68 REVERSE AGIN

BY SCIENCE

HOW TO GET 20 YEARS YOUNGER: FOUNTAIN OF YOUTH FOUND?

Plus: 28 Antiaging Foods & Elixirs

Plus: 15 Breakthrough Discoveries That Will Keep You Forever Young

By Victoria Fairchild Porter

Other Books from the same Publishing House:

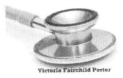

**58 Effective Cancer Therapies
Backed Up By Science
You Probably Never Heard About**

Get Rid Of Any Kind Of Cancer And
Any Other Disease Fast With No Side Effects

Plus: 47 Natural Anti-Cancer Substances

Plus: 12 Controversial/Forbidden Therapies

Victoria Fairchild Porter

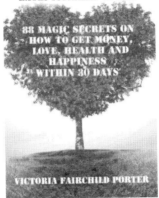

**HOW TO MAKE EVERY DAY
EXCEPTIONALLY LUCKY**

**88 MAGIC SECRETS ON
HOW TO GET MONEY,
LOVE, HEALTH AND
HAPPINESS
WITHIN 30 DAYS**

VICTORIA FAIRCHILD PORTER

222 LOVE TECHNIQUES

**MAKE ANY MAN
FALL IN LOVE WITH YOU**

GET YOUR EX BACK

LEARN THE SECRET LAWS OF ENCHANTMENT

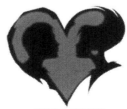

Viktor Parker

Table of Contents

This book is for anyone, who loves life and wants to be young, healthy and beautiful forever because nothing else is more exciting and amazing than life itself in all its forms.

Vanessa Fairchild Parker

September 16, 2016

New York City

It may come as a surprise to many, but yes, it is within your power to make time go backwards and reverse the aging process. You hold the key to turn back your biological clock and the sooner you act on it – the more effective the process will be.

I don't believe in age. People are finally starting to realize that their age is not written in stone, but can be moved in whichever direction they choose to. As many like to say, age is really just a number.

The quest for youth and immortality has always been one of the wildest dreams of humanity. Immortality has been sought throughout the world by millions of both genders. Statistics show that about 100,000 people die each day from aging. Each year over $160 billion are spent on finding the fountain of youth. Lifespan has been driven up for the past century and according to statistics, in 2050 the number of people 60 years or older will be approximately 2 billion, compared to less than a billion today.

Man has long dreamt of cheating death and keeping youth forever and that is about to become a reality soon. Humanity has always fantasized of being able to reverse the aging process and we have never been closer to that moment than today.

"I don't want to achieve immortality through my works. I want to achieve it by not dying". Woody Allen

It appears as though life extending medicine is now coming up with another miracle each day and the time we would be able to live forever is just around the corner – scientists say that it will happen within the next 5-10 years. Until then, your mission should be to grow younger every day.

Homo sapiens will never get used to the idea that he is mortal. So here come the legends of a mythical potion – the elixir of life, which can keep your youth for eternity.

Myths about eternal life have been known since the beginning of time. Some are still in a quest for the Holy Grail – the cup that provides eternal youth, happiness and food in infinite abundance. To make an elixir for an eternal life has been the dream of many scientists throughout the past centuries. In Ancient China many emperors sought the fabled elixir of immortality.

To reverse aging has been the Holy Grail for medicine. One of the ever-present life-long quests of humans results in millions of researchers trying to figure out what can stop and reverse aging. They are studying worms, rats, fruit flies, molecules, etc.

Often the results don't have a happy ending – remember the Chinese Emperor Qin Shi Huang who died after he drank an elixir of immortality?

The history of scientific pursuits keeps for us stories from the Egyptian medical papyrus, Ayurveda followers, Alchemists and Tibetan monks. Ancient Greek sources mention a tree juice, which extends human life and Ancient Indians talk about a tree that extends human life to 10,000 years.

Trees can live a very long time – for example, there are records of a macro zamia tree "Great Grand Father Peter", which is midway between a fern and a palm and which is believed to be 15,000 years old. A California White Mountains bristlecone pine tree is believed to be 5,000 years old and a pine tree in Greece is said to be the oldest tree in Europe – over 1000 years old.

Some animals also live longer than humans – there is a jellyfish, which was discovered in the Mediterranean in the 1880s. It never truly dies, but rather recycles itself while aging backwards from adult stage to an immature polyp stage over and over again. A Greenland shark can live 400 years, a deep sea clam, named after a Chinese dynasty during which it was born, lived for 507 years and was accidentally killed in 2006 while scientists tried to transport it for climate change research.

In Middle Ages alchemists kept on looking for that philosophical stone, which turns metals to gold, cures all diseases and guarantees eternal life.

Nature has invested so much perfection in the creation of any living creature and plant. And man is undoubtedly the most genius creation of all.

The normal life span according to healers should be 154 years (22 stages by 7 years each). According to another rule, a law in biology, mammals live 5-7 times the length of their development. Therefore the human lifespan should be 125-175 years because the period of his development is 25 years.

The Japanese emperor Jimmu is known to have ruled Japan for 126 years. The Greek priest Epimenid somehow managed to extend his life to 300 years. According to Chinese legends, Guan Chen Czi legendary lived for over 1400 years. LP Suwang, who died in 1995 was rumored to be capable of miracles. He lived for 200 years.

Swami Buaji jogi lived in New York and left the city when he was said to be 116 years old. Tao Porchon-Lynch, 98 is an active yoga instructor, who started taking ballroom dancing lessons when she was 90.

In his history of India, Peter Maffens talks about a man named Numise Cogua, who was 370 years old and whose teeth, hair and beard grew 4 times. He died in 1566. Himalayans often live over 120 years in good health.

So many cases have made headlines in terms of female fertility either. You might have read about the 70 year old Rajo Devi Lohan from India, who gave a first time birth to a baby at 70 through IVF, the 72 year old Daljinder Kaur, who gave birth to a healthy boy in April 2016 or Malegwale Ramokgopa, who allegedly gave birth in 1931 to twins 3 days after her 92nd birthday.

Today scientists have ways to change the genomes of embryos and make a child a centenarian before it's even born.

There are cases when people with genetic anomalies start aging too fast and there are cases of people, who start growing backwards once they hit a certain age. An example of that is the sensational case of the Japanese woman Say Senagon from Fukoka, who started getting younger once she turned 75. This happened in the nineties of the last century. Fist her gray hair turned to black. Then her gums started to bleed and she could not wear her dentures – turned out she had new teeth growing. Say started having strong sexual desires, her wrinkles disappeared, her skin became smooth and no one was able to recognize her. She also resumed her menstrual cycle soon after. Say divorced her husband of

50 years and married a 40 year old man. Soon after, she even had a child. People in Japan wanted to know how she regained her youth and there were detectives following her all over who reported what she ate, how she exercised, slept, etc. She later got examined in the Institute of gerontology and it got clear that what caused her unusual aging backwards was a natural process in her body.

The team of scientists discovered a gene – "oncogene", which was able to destroy aged cells. This gene is able under certain circumstances to lead to diseases, and under others – to reverse aging in the human body. Usually, oncogenes lead to uncontrollable cell division and eventually create tumors, but in Say's case – they have somehow acted as genes of youth.

As of now scientists haven't been able to discover the reason of the awakening of the youth gene in Say, but they believe it's possible that the activation may have happened after she had to take a lot of bio-stimulators for her liver surgery.

There is something in our body that can maintain youthfulness and it has been a lifelong quest for many trying to find out where the secret is hidden.

What could be holding the key of the fountain of youth? Is it something inside of us or is it some substance we can source from nature or maybe a procedure?

Your body is able to repair itself if you treat it in a certain way. Your cells require energy and proper nutrition. Your cells die and replace themselves at certain intervals and each cell can be replaced by a weaker cell, the same strength cell or a stronger and better cell. You can be in charge of that process and it's totally up to you to make it happen and regenerate your body to a younger one and I will show you how to do that in this book and you will learn what are the secrets of people who look and feel 30 years younger than their calendar age and how to do it yourself.

Long life however is not that great when you sacrifice the social part of it in order to live long and stop doing many things that you enjoy. Have you noticed that most people want to stay away from individuals who are obsessed with eating in a certain way or being slaves to different extreme diets and rituals. Once you lose the fun part of life, and stop enjoying it, your body stops helping you reverse aging, because your mind doesn't enjoy the process and anything you don't really enjoy doesn't work.

Your chances of reversing aging to an extent that would satisfy you even if you follow the best vegan diet and work out religiously are quite slim. I will introduce you to 68 Therapies, many of which are beyond proper nutrition and exercise. Some of these therapies have been used successfully by many, others - by a few individuals only, but have achieved exceptional results.

This book could have been 50 times longer, while giving you the same amount of actual information at the same time. My purpose is to make sure you learn the maximum amount of information in the most possibly synthetized way without boring you with pages and pages of stories which have no relevance to what you want to know.

I will introduce you to many therapies from all over the world – USA, Russia, Japan, China, etc., designed to reverse aging either naturally, through a pill or through a certain procedure. I will tell you what works and what doesn't work based on the experience of people who have tried it, what the science says about these therapies and what is coming up in the pipeline, which will make you immortal.

Some studies are industry sponsored and less objective, some are not. Many foods have been wrongly demonized in the past, but the newest studies show that they are in fact good for you.

There have been so many studies conducted on almost everything and the more studies come out to life, the more of them simply contradict each other. The University of Harvard for example will conclude that this and that is good, while Stanford University researchers will swear into exactly the opposite outcome. As a result, we all get confused on what is good for us and what is not. Many studies that test groups of people also add other activities to their change of diet like exercise and meditation, which changes the final outcome a lot, because since the diet wasn't the only variable that is different between all groups, then we don't really know whether those good results were due to the diet or to the other techniques.

Take coffee for example. Hundreds of studies show it's good for you and it's full of antioxidants and encourage you to drink it, while hundreds of other teams of scientists and nutritionists claim it's the worst drink you could put inside your body and you should definitely quit it.

Researchers are doing their best to increase the number of healthy years in people's lives and one of the reasons they are now able to extend lifespan is because they can prevent diseases. The better quality of life you have – the harder it would be for any disease to get to you and the longer your life span will be.

Before you start any of the antiaging therapies in this book, you need to stabilize your health first and make sure you have done your best to get rid of any disease within your body. Any pain you have in your body shows up on your face, changes your face expression and makes you look tired and older. Chronic pain and inflammation age you extensively. To learn how to prevent and get rid of almost any man-created disease including cancer, you can find great advices in the book "How to Cure Cancer: 78 Effective Cancer Therapies Backed Up By Science You Probably Never Heard About". This book will teach you how to better take care of your body even if you don't have cancer.

The longer you could keep yourself healthy – the longer you will live. Suppressing disease symptoms by taking drugs is very profitable for the pharmaceutical industry, but it is neither helping your body get rid of the disease, neither sparing you from the multiple side effects of each drug.

If you feel like many bad things are happening to you and you don't know why that might be, what you are doing wrong and how to change that, you will find good explanations in the book "101 Proven Techniques to Overcome Depression and Anxiety".

Disclaimer:

I am unaware of any pre-existing health conditions you might have. You should consult with a qualified medical practitioner before using any of the therapies in this book. The therapies in this book are not meant to be substitute for a sound medical advice. If you have an acute or chronic condition, you should consult your Doctor before using on yourself any of the recommended therapies listed below. The author makes no claims about the effectiveness of the treatments described in this book.

CHAPTER I – THE 7 CAUSES OF AGING ACCORDING TO LEADING US SCIENTISTS PLUS 7 OTHER CAUSES POINTED BY EUROPEAN RESEARCHERS

Scientists have identified several fundamental causes of aging.

What causes aging? There are different opinions - some believe the foods we eat and the sun exposure are the major reasons for aging, others think it's the way we breathe and our genes, but they all agree that everyone's biological age is different from their chronological age and that is due to different lifestyles, habits and diets.

Some scientists believe that the number one cause of aging is glycation, followed by oxidative stress and telomere shortening.

Glycation

When we heat food, it undergoes chemical changes and creates acidic toxins. That's how twisted carbohydrates, fats and proteins are created and also carcinogens, which results in Advanced Glycation End Products (AGEs).

Glucose binds to our proteins, lipids and DNA and they get unable to function properly and cause aging. So the least processed is the food you eat – the better.

Oxidative Stress

Oxidants contain oxygen and are highly reactive substances, which damage the DNA, the fats and the proteins. Free radicals steal energy (electrons). They are called oxidizing (acidic) and they cause decay. Free radicals are missing an electron and are therefore unstable molecules. They are deficient in energy and cause cellular damage (dry, sagging and wrinkled skin).

Free radicals are the culprits for our aging. They attack healthy molecules, steal their electrons and create new free radicals. The way to stop this process is to take anti-oxidants, which have spare electrons and therefore an excess of energy, which it gives up in favor of the free radicals and neutralizes them.

Avoid drinking, smoking, radiation, stress, coffee, polluted air and processed foods as much as possible in order to avoid the above sources of free radicals.

Healthy food does the opposite – it alkalizes your body or contributes energy (electrons), and such foods have high Oxygen Radical Absorbance Capacity. The ones that are high in beta-carotene, lycopene and chlorophyll are the best for you. Such are fruits, vegetables, raw sprouts, herbs, spices and nuts.

There are no antioxidants in meat, fish, eggs and diary.

Sadly, feeding laboratory mice with anti-oxidants haven't shown so far that it extends their lives and according to some theories, free radicals might even be somewhat beneficial. For example, when scientists gave anti-oxidants to a worm, it had a negative impact on its lifespan.

Telomere shortening

Telomeres are sequences of nucleotides at the ends of chromosomes, which protect the ends of chromosomes from fusion with other chromosomes or from deterioration. Every time a cell replicates itself, the telomeres get shorter and this eventually leads to cellular damage. This happens with a different rate with different people, as factors which contribute to this are both genetic and due to lifestyle.

An enzyme has been discovered, called telomerase, which can reverse the telomere shortening and it is found in the human body as well as in certain plants.

However, some scientists like Aubrey de Grey, who is one of the leading researchers in the world in the field of biomedical gerontology, believe that telomere shortening is actually playing a minor role in aging.

Membrane Damage

DNA Damage

Inflammation

Chronological age is the last factor and the one that plays the smallest role in our aging.

According to scientists, chronological age and genetics play a small role in our aging – only 6%. Genes you have inherited do matter to a certain extent, but your lifestyle and your diet matters way more.

According to Aubrey de Grey, there are 7 causes of aging and his team is experimenting with therapies that can fix those causes:

1. **Loss of cells in tissues** – can be fixed through cell therapy;

2. **Accumulation of extra cellular junks** – can be fixed through phagocytosis by immune stimulation;

3. **Accumulation of mutations responsible for cancer** – can be fixed through telomerase gene deletion plus periodic stem cell reseeding;

4. **Mutations in the Mitochondria** (organelles found in large numbers in most cells, in which the biochemical processes of energy production and respiration occur) –

can be fixed through allotropic expression of 13 proteins. According to latest theories, if you stop mitochondrial damage early enough – it is also reversible;

5. **Accumulation of indigestible molecules** (inside the cells) – causes atherosclerosis – can be fixed through transgenic microbial hydrolases;

6. **Death–resistant cells** – can be fixed through suicide genes and immune stimulation;

7. **Accumulation of cross-links** – can be fixed through AGE – breaking molecules/enzymes.

Aubrey de Gray believes that if we are able to clean our bodies of all the junk inside, we will reduce the mutations in our mitochondria and will also be able to stop hydrogen peroxide, which is a free radical released by mitochondria. Hydrogen peroxide is the main cause of the oxidation of our bodies.

CHAPTER II – HOW TO REVERSE AGING

Your body is created infinitely wise, by design and is programmed to be healthy.

You have to accept and believe that the default state of your body is the state of ceaseless regeneration.

When it comes to foods and nutrition, the "What doesn't kill you makes you stronger" rule does not apply. Some foods or food combinations you eat will kill you but slowly, in a way that you wouldn't even notice.

I will start in the beginning with therapies that we all know, but very few of us actually practice. It is always good to re-affirm and remind ourselves that those are the things that really work and can make us younger.

Therapy 1: NEVER COMBINE PROTEINS WITH SUGAR AVOID ALL FORMS OF SUGAR, INCLUDING GRAINS

Why? Because it creates Advanced Glycation End products (AGEs) which age you fast.

When sugars in your body attach to the proteins and amino acids, they create sugar proteins or Advanced Glycation End Products (AGEs), which process ages you. This can occur both in the food that you eat and inside your body. We have a lot of sugars and proteins naturally flowing in our bodies and they create this chemical reaction when together. Even though glucose is a necessary fuel for our body, when we have too much of it, along with oxidation - it is damaging to us. Glycation is in a way a "caramelization" of our tissues and declining of organ functioning.

Refined sugar causes fatty liver, diabetes, obesity and heart disease.

The problem with sugar is that it is everywhere – in your glass of wine, in your ketchup, French fries, etc. Sugar is stored as a fat, unless your body uses it immediately for energy. The excess sugar attaches to collagen and causes wrinkles on your skin. Your body produces antibodies to AGEs since it doesn't recognize them as natural parts of your body and that is how inflammation in the skin is created. AGEs gravitate towards elastin and collagen and create wrinkles.

According to Bryan Clement, the Director of the Hippocrates Institute in Florida, combining of sugar with proteins of all kinds (which causes glycation) is the number one cause of premature aging along with free radical damage (caused by glycation).

AGEs make your cells more susceptible to damage and premature aging. They are especially high in the animal foods like red meat.

The sugary processed foods are also very high in AGEs. Processed refined sugars don't contain minerals, vitamins or fiber – they are "empty calories" because they have no nutritional value.

Glycation is caused by excess sugar, high temperature cooking, lack of anti-oxidants and excess of carbohydrates. Of all the molecules, damaging your body, the sugar molecules (especially fructose) are the most damaging of all.

Studies show that when AGEs are restricted, it leads to significant increasing of the lifespan.

Foods, containing FRUCTOSE:

Blackberries, bananas, kiwis, mangoes, cherries, figs, mandarins, grapefruits, pineapples, pomegranates, dark plums, apples, pears, raspberries and rockmelon.

Glycation creates inflammation and affects your immune system. Your total fructose consumption shall be below 15-25 grams/day.

Below is the sugar content of a few fruits:

1 apple: 23 grams

1 banana: 17 g.

1 peach: 15 g.

1 serving of Red Grapes: 20 g.

1 serving of cantaloupe: 13 g.

1 serving of water melon: 18 g.

1 serving of orange: 23 g.

1 serving of strawberries: 7 g.

1 serving of pineapple: 9 g.

Glucose:

Your body processes different sugars in a different way. For example, fructose is much worse for you than glucose as when you eat fructose, you put on much more weight than when you eat glucose. Every cell in your body and your brain feeds with glucose and glucose is not as big of a burden to the liver as the fructose is. Fructose is stored as fat, instead of burned up the way glucose is.

Since your body utilizes glucose, it gets burned up shortly after consumption, while fructose gets converted to fatty acids, cholesterol and fat. Glucose suppresses your appetite. Grapes and honey have very high glucose contents.

Vegetables contain starch (chains of glucose linked together), which is their energy storage molecule. Some vegetables like zucchini, squash and corn are high in starch contents and others like eggplant, mushrooms, cabbage, cucumbers, green beans, tomatoes, green peppers and asparagus have low contents of starch.

Fructose is largely converted into fat unlike glucose, which stores less than 1% of the calories you eat as fat. Once fructose is metabolized, large part of it is converted to uric acid and toxins, which cause the weight gain process.

Agave syrup is not good for you contrary to the wide spread beliefs, because once processed, the nutritional benefits of the agave plant are reduced to almost nothing and the syrup itself contains almost all fructose.

Since sugar is very addictive, it is really difficult to cut it all together, but artificial sweeteners are even worse for you than fructose, so avoid them at any rate.

Therapy 2: CONSUME LESS REFINED CARBS

Refined carbs are hidden sugars. Many carbs, such as pasta, white bread and cookies also break down to sugar in your body. Carbs destroy your leptin and insulin sensitivity and lead to premature aging.

Starches turn into sugar once they reach your bloodstream. The levels of sugar in your blood soar and your pancreas releases insulin in your bloodstream to help your cells convert the glucose into cell fuel. However, the body usually releases too much insulin, your sugar blood levels drop and you get hungry again very soon after.

Refined carbs are plant based foods and have their whole grain extracted during processing like most breakfast cereals, breads, all desserts, cookies, crackers, candy, pasta, bagels, pizza, pancakes, white rice, sugar, white potatoes, French fries, cookies, maple syrup, etc. During refining the fiber is removed as well as their nutrients. These foods break down into sugar and have a very high glycemic index and they create inflammation, which makes you look older. Your body produces high levels of insulin after eating of such foods.

All processed foods are high in harmful ingredients and chemical additives, artificial chemicals and are low in nutritional contents.

Solution: Eat complex carbohydrates instead like vegetables, legumes and whole grains – it takes longer for the body to digest them and the sugar gets released slower.

Therapy 3: CHANGE YOUR COOKING METHODS OR JUST MODIFY THEM A LITTLE BIT

Why? Because once you grill or roast the meat, you create additional amount of Advanced Glycation End products (AGEs).

Your body has mechanisms to eliminate AGEs, but once they become too many – it can't get rid of them effectively. Once AGEs start accumulating in your body, it creates many chronic diseases.

Scientists advise that a diet low in AGEs is necessary if you want to get the AGEs circulating in your body out of your system and especially if you have diabetes, since AGEs have been said to be a potential cause for diabetes. Studies show that diabetes patients who reduced the AGEs in their diet, improved their hyperinsulinemia by about 40%.

Dry heat promotes AGE formation. Meats that are high in protein and fats are very likely to form AGEs during cooking, opposite to fruits, vegetables and whole grains, which have low levels of AGE after cooking.

You can measure the levels of AGE in your body with AGE scanner, which uses LED light to penetrate your skin.

Solution: Cook shorter, use moist heat (steamed or boiled) instead of dry heat, use lower temperatures and use lemon or vinegar, which acidic properties reduce AGE levels. Cook in a slow cooker. It's better to cook your food a bit longer on a low heat, than shorter at a higher heat. Eat more fruits and vegetables. For example noni, blueberries and cranberries were found to have iridoids, which can lower AGE levels in your body. Sleep more – while your body sleeps, it reduces the levels of AGEs.

Therapy 4: IMMORTALITY HERBS

Here are some herbs that are used to extend the health life span in the traditional Indian medicine Ayurveda and in Chinese medicine and are known as immortality herbs:

Rasayanas: Ocimum sanctum, Bacopa monnieri, Curcuma longa, Centella asiatica, Phyllanthus emblica, Withania somnifera, Chinese tea Jiaogulan.

Other herbs are Astragalus, Reishi, Cordyceps and Schizandra. These are the herbs that have been taken daily by yogis and Tibetan monks, who lived way over 100 years.

CHAPTER III – AVOID THESE FOODS. THEY ARE THE BIGGEST CULPRITS FOR PREMATURE AGING

Therapy 5: DON'T EAT FOODS THAT CAUSE DEGENERATION AND AGE YOU

You are aging from inside out and the main culprit for that are the foods you eat. Some foods have the ability to accelerate the aging process and make you look and feel older.

Processed Meats

Processed meats are hot dogs, bacon, salami, etc. and they contain sulfates, nitrates, and a lot of preservatives, salt and are high in saturated fats. They can create inflammation and contribute to aging.

Heated oil

All fried foods like French fries, fried eggs, fried meat and fish age you. When oil is exposed to high temperatures, the oil gets unstable, high temperatures cause oxidation in the oil and once it gets into the human body, it causes inflammation.

Cook with organic virgin coconut or grape seed oil instead.

Use organic extra virgin olive oil on your salads.

Trans-fat Foods

Trans-fats are manufactured fats, as the manufacturers add hydrogen to vegetable oil and that's how oil becomes solid when at room temperature. For example, margarine is a trans-fat. Most of crackers, potato chips, cookies, microwave popcorn and frozen pizzas contain trans-fats. FDA has now banned all trans-fats in 2015 and manufacturers have been given 3 years to comply. The deadline for all trans-fats to be eliminated from foods is 2018. Trans-fats lower your good cholesterol and raise your bad one. If your body is contaminated with build-up of trans-fats, you will never get the chance to lose weight no matter how much you try.

Dairy Products in Large Amounts

Studies show that approximately 60% of adults are not able to digest dairy products, which ends up creating inflammation in their bodies. Dairy has also been linked to acne and other problematic skin conditions like age spots. Dairy also contains a protein, which causes irritation and inflammation in your joints and it might contribute to arthritis. Milk has been also proven to deplete the calcium from your bones.

Salt

You only need about ¾ of a teaspoon of salt a day so your body functions properly. Any extra amount creates inflammation in your joints, dehydrates you and can lead to high blood pressure and kidney disease.

Best salt to use is pink Himalayan salt.

Alcohol

Alcohol creates inflammation. If you drink it occasionally, it will not hurt you much, but once it gets a regular habit – it will age you a lot. Alcohol breaks down to sugar and accelerates aging. Alcohol ruins your liver, which has an important function to detoxify your body. Alcohol ruins your skin - it dehydrates you, which causes the skin to create more wrinkles. It triggers many skin conditions like inflammation, breakouts, redness and sensitivity because your blood vessels dilate due to alcohol. Your skin will look tired and dry.

You also know that alcohol doesn't let you sleep well. You will fall asleep, but will wake up in the middle of the night from the sugar rush.

The more contents of sugar the alcohol you consume has – the more it ages you.

Soda

No two opinions here – it's definitely bad for you. It contains sugar or artificial sweeteners, both of which are bad for you. Artificial sweeteners cause inflammation.

Coffee

Coffee has many benefits as it is full of anti-oxidants and it improves your concentration, mood, short term memory and it really wakes you up. Some studies even show it may reduce your risk of skin cancer.

The bad side of coffee is that it dehydrates you, stains your teeth and has high amounts of caffeine, which can get you shaken if you have too much of it. I have a friend who believes that Starbucks adds certain additives to their coffee, which makes you get addicted. I don't know if they do so, but caffeine by itself is extremely addictive for your brain and I felt the withdrawal symptoms on myself after I decided to quit coffee after many years of drinking it – I had headaches daily for 2-3 months from the caffeine withdrawal effect.

Chaga is a very good substitute of coffee and is good for you. Just rinse your mouth after you are finished drinking it, because it can stain your teeth even worse than coffee.

Processed foods - dead food makes you age prematurely and creates diseases.

Genetically modified foods create genetic changes in your body. Those foods are carriers of distorted information fields.

Oysters and mussels - they eat sea garbage.

Artificial sweeteners and additives

Preservatives

CHAPTER IV – SUPERFOODS THAT CAN MAKE YOU DECADES YOUNGER

Therapy 6: TAKE ANTI-OXIDANTS. BEST WAY IS TO GET YOUR ANTI-OXIDANTS FROM FOOD

According to the free radical theory, you should take anti-oxidant supplements like Vitamin C, Q10, Carnosine, Lipoic acid, N-acetylcysteine and Vitamin E, which do extend human life. However, there are clinical trials made on vitamin E (high doses intake) and beta carotene, which suggest that those supplements actually increase mortality rates.

Obviously, the more antioxidants a food has, the better it can work to reverse aging. For example, good sources of antioxidants are the foods below:

Eat the following anti-aging foods with high oxygen radical absorbance capacity (ORAC) value:

	ORAC VALUE
Spices	314,446
Oregano dried	200,129
Chaga mushrooms	110,400
Acai berries	102,700
Goji berries	25,300
Beans	8,000
Pistachio nuts	7,983
Plums	7,581
Blueberries	6,552
Blackberries	5,347
Garlic (raw)	5,346
Cilantro	5,141
Raspberries	4,882

EAT SUPERFOODS BLUE-GREEN ALGAE, SPIRULINA AND CHLORELLA.

Sprouts together with spirulina, chlorella and the blue-green algae are the most nutritious foods in existence.

28

In our bodies there are hundreds of different chemical reactions going on at any time and it needs at least 90 different vitamins, minerals and fatty acids to ensure its proper functions.

SUPERFOODS THAT MAKE YOU 10 YEARS YOUNGER:

The superfoods are natural organic foods, which have high concentration of antioxidants, nutrients, enzymes and amino-acids. There are many studies done on these foods and they all confirm the extremely beneficial properties they have on our health. These foods were found to have more digestible protein than beef, 11 times more calcium than a cup of cow's milk, they can boost your metabolism and eventually reverse the aging of your body.

Below are the healthiest foods that can make you younger if you consume them regularly.

Seaweeds also soak up fat from your body. Scientists from Newcastle University in UK discovered that seaweeds have chemical properties that prevent the fat from being digested by your body. Once you add them to your diet, not only will you feel the anti-aging but also the slimming effect of this amazing food.

Chlorella

Chlorella is a green algae, which has been a subject of thousands of studies in Taiwan and Japan. It contains vitamins A, B (has more vitamin B12 than liver), C, E, D, K, beta carotene, lutein, minerals (like magnesium and zink), 18 amino acids and other nutrients. Chlorella boosts metabolism, clobbers abnormal cell growth, regulates cholesterol levels in the body and can make you decades younger.

It helps blood carry oxygen throughout the body and neutralizes the environmental toxins.

Chlorella is very popular in Japan and people who take it regularly are healthy even in their 90's.

Spirulina

Spirulina is also a green algae, which contains a very high concentration of protein by weight – much more than any other known food so far. It also contains vitamins B, E, K, beta carotene, iron, magnesium and essential fatty acids (good fats), which can keep your brain and heart healthy. Spirulina gives you energy and promotes a healthy immune system.

Barley Grass

Barley grass is rich in antioxidants and nutrients and can detoxify your liver and protect your cells from damage.

Barley is rich in fiber and helps clean your colon. It changes the acidity of your body to alkaline, contains more iron than spinach, more calcium than milk and more vitamin C than citrus fruits.

Wheatgrass Juice

Try this elixir of life and your dark circles will disappear and your grey hair will turn back with time.

Royal Jelly

Royal jelly is known as a super food, which has anti-aging properties and it can help beat many diseases including depression.

It is full of nutrients and zink, iron, vitamins A, B complex, C, D, E, folic acid, calcium, amino acids and collagen. That's why it's so good for your skin when taken both internally and externally.

Royal jelly is also able to enhance your blood circulation.

Turmeric and Golden Milk drink

Studies show that if you add only 1 gram of turmeric to your breakfast, it could improve your memory.

Many of you know a drink called "golden milk" became very popular recently. It is made from turmeric and black pepper.

A study shows that if one adds 20grams of black pepper (with active ingredient piperine) to the curcumin, its bioavailability increase by 2000%. The same way, when you eat apples (their skin contains quercentin) together with dark chocolate, rich in flavonoids, you boost their benefits and they act in a much more powerful way.

Turmeric contains curcumin, which has anti-inflammatory, anti-oxidant and anti-cancer properties. It boosts the immune system, detoxifies the liver, promotes good brain function, regulates the metabolism and helps to maintain the cholesterol levels.

Mix ¼ cup of turmeric with half spoon of black pepper and a cup of bottled water. Stir until the mixture becomes a paste. Part 2: take 1 cup of milk (soy, almond, etc.) and 1 tea spoon of coconut oil and add ¼ teaspoon of the previously made turmeric paste. Heat and stir without allowing it to boil. Once ready, add some honey and enjoy!

Fruits and vegetables that reverse the signs of aging. eat the following foods which help regeneration and have anti-aging effect:

Honey, Bee Pollen, Cinnamon, Acai, Berries, Garlic, Avocado, Unprocessed Rice (Brown Rice soaked for approx.. 20 hours), Quinoa, Sauerkraut, Cabbage, Sprouts, Beans, Oat meal, Greens, Ginger, Nuts, Yogurt, Potatoes, Melons, Chaga, Cacao, Beets, Essiac Tea, Maca, Maqui, Coconuts, Mangosteen, Longan, Flax seed oil, Goji berries, Stevia (tiny bit), Amino acids (apple vinegar, lemon juice), Sulfur rich foods (Beans – soak them for approximately 8 hours, which will make them alkaline. This is how they get sprouted, Soy, Tofu, Onions, Garlic); Egg yolks; Tomatoes; Fulvic acid, Macao, Burdock, Ginger, Coriander, Cilantro, Noni, Red clover, Cordyceps, Chia, foods rich in omega 4 & 5 fatty acids (evening primrose, fish oil), Licorice (stimulates the regeneration of the liver), Broccoli is loaded with nutrients, Raw nuts.

Blueberries

According to a study conducted in 2010, blueberries when combines with carnosine (found in milk, eggs, cheese, beef, poultry and pork) and green tea regenerate stem cells in animal models.

They will keep your memory sharp and your complexion great because they are full of vitamin C.

Blueberries are packed with antioxidants and they can fight the free radicals, which damage your skin and organ cells.

Elderly people who were a subject to a study were given 2 cups of blueberries a day for 6 weeks and their mobility improved significantly after.

Pomegranate

Pomegranate contains polyphenol, which can inhibit inflammation in brain cells. This fruit is an elixir of youth and delays aging.

Avocado

Studies show that avocado oil can affect the mitochondria in a way that it can lower the production of damaging free radicals.

Avocados contain a lot of antioxidants, which protect against free radicals and can reverse aging. They are full of healthy raw fats and they contain nearly all essential nutrients that our bodies are not able to produce on their own. The nutrients from avocados can activate the energy production of the mitochondria.

They also have antifungal and antibacterial properties, promote a healthy immune system and boost brain activity.

Avocado oil can soften your skin, boost collagen and reduce aging spots when used externally.

Cocoa and Dark Chocolate

As you know, dark chocolate has longevity benefits due to the cocoa which it is made of. The latest evidence suggests that dark chocolate prevents white blood cells from sticking to the walls of blood vessels and helps restore flexibility to arteries. It has been found to deter atherosclerosis. There are naturally occurring bio actives in cocoa - flavanols, which help reverse the age related memory problems. Lavado cocoa extract helps preventing Alzheimer's disease. Also cocoa flavanols may lower inflammation, boost brain power and keep blood pressure normal.

Coconut water has the same level of electrolytic balance as human blood, so it is very good for you. It is lower in sugars and salts than other drinks and higher in potassium.

Eat dark chocolate with high percentage of cocoa powder. Choose one that has 85 % or higher cocoa contents. Dark chocolate has been proven to deliver health benefits like anti-inflammatory effect on your cells, reduce blood pressure, improve your mood and prevent certain types of cancer like colon cancer.

Don't eat chocolate close to bed time, because it will keep you awake.

Raw Seeds and Soaked and Sprouted Grains

Seeds and raw nuts should be sprouted to neutralize their enzyme inhibitor and phytic acid. Otherwise the above substances would inhibit our own enzymes and will stop the absorption of iron, zink, copper and calcium. Sprouting breaks down the starch and makes inactive the toxic ingredients which may exist in them. Soaking/sprouting releases enzymes like papain and protease.

Sprouting releases dormant vitamins, minerals, proteins, fats and carbohydrates. They are alkalizing to your body.

Tomatoes

Tomatoes are very good for you. They are rich in lycopene – a powerful antioxidant, which can keep your skin smooth and protect you from sunburn. Studies have been made with tomatoes which show that once cooked, the content of vitamin C decreases by up to 29%, but the trans-lycopene content of the cooked tomatoes on the opposite – increases by up to 164%.

Kale

Kale contains a lot of vitamin K, fiber and nutrients.

Red Bell Peppers

They are full of Vitamin C, which fights wrinkles because it promotes the production of collagen and fights bacteria and germ in your body.

Mango

Mango is full of Vitamins A, B, C, beta-carotene and Omega-3 fatty acids.

Mangosteen

Mangosteen has powerful antifungal, anti-inflammatory, antiseptic and antimicrobial properties.

Spinach and dark greens will make your vision sharp. They are rich in vitamin K, which can reduce bone loss.

Yogurt

The probiotics in yogurt are very good for you and they can ensure a lower risk of tooth loss and gum disease.

Beet juice

Beet juice is a nitrate-rich drink and has been proven to be an endurance booster – according to scientists from the University of Exeter, it helps you exercise up to 16% longer. It also improves decision making during games like football.

Yams

Yams are an excellent antiaging food. Eat them preferably raw by juicing them or blending them.

Nuts

Studies show that nuts are filling and help you eat less. Turns out that up to 20 percent of the calories they contain don't get absorbed.

Green Tea

Many studies show that green tea protects against DNA damage, oxidative stress, inflammation and depression. Green tea also promotes bone health or fights osteoporosis.

A study of 2009 found that the active compound in green tea – EGCG extends the life of round worms. EGCG also has the ability to produce stress-producing proteins.

Rats, which were given green tea supplements lived on the average of 14% longer than the rest of the rats.

A study of Campbell University shows that people in Japan who practice a green tea ceremony live longer than average.

A study of 2010 concludes that green tea may delay the signs of skin aging – wrinkles and sun damage.

Coconut Oil

Cook with coconut oil and do regular oil pulling with coconut oil. Coconut oil is an excellent anti-aging food and it's good for you to both eat it as well as apply it on your skin as a moisturizer. According to Brian Clement, the Director of Hippocrates Institute in Florida, it is best for external purposes.

Omega – 3 fish oil and Omega – 3 rich fish

Take more Omega – 3 fats, such as natural fish oil or krill oil (take 500 mg/day) fats and less Omega 6 fats (trans-fats).

Omega – 3 protects against inflammation in the brain cells and leads to improved mood. Flaxseed, walnuts, salmon and tuna have anti-inflammatory effect on human body.

Flaxseed oil is believed to be the richest vegetable source of Omega-3 fatty acids, which are very important for your skin to stay lubricated.

Omega 7

The tests results on animal models have been remarkable. Omega-7 can reduce blood lipid levels and improve insulin sensitivity. It turns out to be able to fight and maybe reverse inflammatory changes caused by obesity.

Amino Acids

Each time your body lacks amino acids, it takes them from your skin's collagen and your skin starts looking old. Two amino acids are most important for the construction of your connective tissues - **glycine and proline**. Foods high in amino acids are soy, beef, tofu, chicken, eggs, milk and cottage cheese.

Your skin needs **Cysteine** in order to stay elastic, protected from outside elements and healthy. Rich in cysteine are egg yolks, beans, soya, garlic and onion.

CHAPTER V – WHICH EATING HABITS AGE YOU MOST AND WHY YOU HAVE TO CHANGE THEM ONCE AND FOREVER

Therapy 7: FOLLOW THESE EATING RULES:

According to Dr. Bryant Clement, it's not good to **eat before 11am and after 11 pm**, because your body cleanses overnight.

Take antioxidants at night, when your body needs them to rejuvenate. During the day, your body produces them.

Eat simple foods. Living foods can rejuvenate your DNA. When you eat simple foods like fruits and vegetables, it is easier for your body to digest them. The more processed a food is – the harder it is to digest it.

Make sure you eat different foods and can give your body the variety of nutrients it needs if you want to start reversing the aging process.

What to eat: Eat a healthy whole plant based food diet with ideally organic foods and at least 70% raw foods – fruits and vegetables.

Concentrate on the taste of the food while chewing it – that brings Prana to your body because you are taking the energy of the food you are chewing. **Chew it slowly**. When you concentrate on the taste of the food, your brain makes your body produce the necessary ferments which your stomach needs to digest the food and take out the minerals, vitamins & nutrients out of it.

Always eat fruits that are in season. When you eat local fruits that are in season you get your body feel better connected with nature, but what really matters a lot is that you will eat them while they are fresh.

Make sure you get enough vitamin B12. B12 deficiency is one of the main reasons for aging. Your skin will get wrinkled if you lack it. Eat beef liver if you want to get it in a natural way.

Never overcook your food.

Try muscle testing to figure out what foods are good for you. You might think what you eat is good for you, but unless you do an actual muscle testing, you have no way to know for sure. You should avoid foods that cause degeneration.

CHAPTER VI - CONTROVERSIAL FOODS - ARE THEY GOOD OR BAD FOR YOU? SHOULD YOU BE VEGETARIAN OR NOT? VEGAN OR NOT?

The first modern vegetarian we know of was the Greek mathematician and philosopher Pythagoras.

About Animal Proteins. Should You Eat Meat Or Not?

Many studies conclude that animal protein is harmful. Others, on the contrary, say that animal protein helps people gain muscle, increases fat burning, reduces appetite, lowers blood pressure, reduces symptoms of diabetes and improves bone health. The "China Study" book by biochemist T. Colin Campbell makes a case that animal foods are the main cause of diseases like cancer and heart disease and which is supported by a study called the China-Cornell-Oxford Project. However, the book has been criticized by many authors who further analyzed the results of the study, not to mention those results have been contradicted by many other studies.

And no, you are not what you eat! You are not a chicken and you are not kale. You are a human being and human beings are different and their bodies have different feels and needs. Some feel better when they eat meat, some when they don't.

Some people who switch to a vegan diet begin having unhealthy look, because they lose their face fat and they start looking older instead of younger.

About the moral side - yes, it is bad to kill animals in order to eat them, but plants have feelings as well and it has been proven in many studies that they get happy when you water them and sad when you forget to do so. Vegetables are probably not very happy when you eat them.

And of course, the meat we can buy is contaminated with all kinds of pollutants, including antibiotics. So if you eat meat, it should be meat from grass fed animals only.

Raw meat contains L-carnosine, which has been proven to reverse aging.

Also, vegans have to take vitamin B12 in order to function properly though there are exceptions from that rule, which I will mention in a bit.

If you are vegan, have in mind that most vegetarians and vegans have certain nutrient deficiencies:

Vegetarians are iron deficient;

83% of vegans are deficient in Vitamin B12;

Vitamin D levels are 74% lower in vegans;

Vegans have 59% lower levels of DHA and 53% lower levels of EPA.

My personal recommendation: If you are a happy vegan – continue being a vegan. If you are vegetarian and it makes you feel great – good for you! There are also people, who have been on a vegan diet for years and who got back to eating meat because they realized vegan lifestyle is not for them. They feel better and have more energy when they eat meat. If you eat too much meat though – it's definitely better to reduce the amount of meat you eat, but there are really no rules – some people feel and look great when they eat meat every day like Dwayne Johnson for example.

His diet and regimen for 6 months while he was shooting the movie "Hercules" are not for everyone. Dwayne eats meat twice a day, fish once a day, 2 whole eggs 6-8 egg whites, rice, potato, salad and oatmeal. He exercises for 90 minutes a day and he feels and looks great. Dwayne has been living like this for a long time and hasn't eaten a candy since 1989. He is now 44 years old and looks like he could be at any age between 30 and 44.

Raquel Welch also eats regularly meat and fish and looks 30 years younger.

Hitler was vegan, but that didn't make him a better person than other people who eat meat.

So the best thing to do is to just stop judging the ones who have a different diet from yours and be happy with whatever way of eating feels right for you.

You need protein and I am not telling you something new here, but what you might not know is that if you don't get enough protein, it is not bad only for your muscle mass, but also calcium is not able to build your bones. So whether you take it from animal sources or from plants, just make sure you get enough of it.

About Saturated Fats

"No diet will remove all the fat from your body because the brain is entirely fat. Without a brain you might look good, but all you could do is run for public office." - George Bernard Shaw

Fat doesn't actually make you fat. The inability to burn it makes you fat. In order to make your body process fat the right way, you need to fix the receptors of your hormones, and in order to do so, you need to fix the cell membranes. The receptors of the cell membrane need fat – cholesterol and saturated fats.

Saturated fats are butter, cheese, milk, beef, lamb, veal, pork, chicken skin, etc.

You need grass fed butter, meat or cheese in order to make sure your hormones function properly.

Saturated fats are not as bad as trans-fats and are even good in small amounts for people who are active and exercise.

Recent studies confirm that eating a lot of saturated fats is not healthy. Dr. Kevo in Woolard from the imperial College of London has recently conducted a study on mice, which were fed with foods with high amounts of saturated fats. The results of the study showed that the high amount of saturated fats in the blood causes inflammation and tissue damage. If that happens occasionally, it's not a big problem, but if you eat those on a regular basis, it can cause serious problems in your body.

Saturated fats and cholesterol can improve the blood cholesterol and can be good for you. They raise the good cholesterol, which protects you from heart disease. It has been recently found that there is absolutely no association between heart disease and saturated fat consumption. Many studies show that they are actually harmless for the majority of people.

Some people actually feel miserable and have skin problems when on a low fat diet and they feel great when they start eating butter and other saturated fats - their skin improves and they feel better and have more energy.

In conclusion - eating a lot of saturated fats ages you, but eating none of them ages you as well. I can't tell you what exact amount is good for you, because that varies from person to person, but check your blood and consult with your doctor.

About Eggs

If you are vegan and don't eat eggs, I will not try to convince you to start eating them. Just do whatever makes you feel good and whatever you believe is better for you. There are many controversial opinions on whether one should eat eggs or not.

Tibetan monks, who live 140 years and longer, claim that eggs and especially egg yolks are good for you and I personally have no reason to doubt them. Tibetan lamas eat yolks every day and egg whites only after they exercise, because the egg whites they believe can be absorbed only then. Of course, if you eat eggs, you should only eat organic eggs.

Eggs were recently found to raise the level of cholesterol in your blood by only 2%. One egg yolk contains half of the elements which our brain, internal organs and nerves need daily to function properly.

There are many studies on eggs and some of them find eggs extremely harmful because of the cholesterol, others conclude that eggs are very good for you and some studies claim that there is no connection between heart disease and eating eggs. It has recently been proven that many people who get heart attacks have low or normal cholesterol.

CHAPTER VII - PROPER FOOD COMBINING – IS IT NONSENSE OR COULD IT MAKE YOU DECADES YOUNGER?

Therapy 8: PROPER FOOD COMBINING CAN MAKE YOU LOOK AND FEEL AT LEAST A DECADE YOUNGER. TRUE OR FALSE?

Dr. Wayne Pickering is very well known for his food combining program and he does look much younger than his calendar age.

The major reason for your upset stomach, heartburn and flatulence is improper food combining according to many experts. And when your body does not digest the food properly – you are not getting good nutrition.

Food breaks down in your mouth, then in your stomach and finally in your small intestine. You digest mechanically first – by chewing. That is why it is so important to chew well.

A chemical digestion of the food happens in your stomach.

There are 3 basic categories of foods: proteins, carbohydrates and fats.

Proteins break down in your stomach and they require a very high acidic enzyme – pepsin. Carbohydrates are divided into fruits and starches (starchy vegetables like potatoes and corn, breads and grains and beans and other legumes). Fruits pass through your digestive system quickly, but starches require 3 levels of breakdown starting in your mouth, where they should be chewed very well.

If you mix proteins with starches, proteins require a very strong acid to break down and starches require an alkaline digestive medium. When you mix them together – they neutralize and don't digest.

So never eat proteins and starches together, but rather wait two hours after eating protein to eat starch.

Don't eat fruits and vegetables together because fruits break mechanically in your stomach, but they break up chemically in your small intestine. Starches break down in 3 stages, starting in your mouth.

Don't eat desert in the end of your meal. It gets trapped in your stomach with the rest of the food, since it's not digested there. Eat fruits 30-60 minutes before your other meals.

Don't eat lemon and bananas together and don't eat melon in combination with other foods, but just eat it alone by itself.

Tomatoes are a fruit-vegetable like eggplant, zucchini, cucumbers, okra and bell papers and they go very well together.

It is also recommended that you eat fruits in the morning in large amount, have more complex but smaller amount food for lunch and most concentrated food (like proteins) in the least amount in the evening.

Should you mix fruits and vegetables in your smoothie – while it is better not to mix them and have a smoothie of fruits or vegetables only, adding a fruit to your vegetable smoothie makes it tastier and many people are more likely to go through the trouble of preparing it once they know they will enjoy it better.

The above food combining program however, is being called by some "old", "outdated" and "nonsense", because they claim that carbs and proteins are being broken down by specific digestive enzymes, which enzymes don't interfere with each other. They also claim that carbs prevent the use of protein for energy purposes. Same authors also argue that fruits and vegetables are very compatible when in the same meal.

I don't know whether the above is true and I couldn't find any scientific studies being done on this matter, but I know that people who follow the food combining system described above look amazing and decades younger. Raquel Welch for example practices food combining diet and she looks ageless at 73. Tibetan lamas and yogi also advice eating the least possible products at one meal and that is how they do it themselves (they eat one type of product per meal). They live over 120 and look younger than their actual age. On the other hand, there are those who don't follow it and still live to 121. One thing is for sure – if you follow the proper food combining – it will not harm you for sure.

CHAPTER VIII – ANTI-AGING DIET PLANS

When it comes to diet, there are always general guidelines, but there is no one way to eat right for everyone.

Diet low in methionine extends your lifespan

According to researchers, a diet low in methionine can extend your lifespan and make you younger. Methionine is an essential amino acid which can prevent from hair loss, can strengthen your nails and help create cartilage. If you are deficient in methionine, you may get liver inflammation, but if you have too much of it, that will shorten your lifespan and increase your risk of cancer.

Tests in animal models showed that methionine restriction significantly slows down aging and increases lifespan.

Here are the foods that contain methionine: meat, fish, Brazil nuts, parmesan cheese, shellfish, soybeans, eggs, dairy and beans.

Paleo Diet

The Paleo diet has been very popular recently because it consists of whole unprocessed foods coming from nature – foods that our ancestors ate for centuries.

Many people claim this diet has helped them get rid of diseases like cancer and improve their health.

<u>While on a Paleo diet you are allowed to eat</u>: fruits, vegetables, eggs, meat, fish, herbs, nuts, seeds, spices, oils and healthy fats. You are encourages to eat potatoes, sweet potatoes and yams. Eat organic and grass-fed pasture raised if possible.

<u>You have to avoid</u>: Sugar, all processed foods, soft drinks, most dairy products (avoid low fat products), grains (breads, pastas), legumes (beans, lentils, etc.), artificial sweeteners, vegetable oils (soybean, sunflower, grapeseed, etc.) and trans-fats.

Rainbow diet

Eat colorful fruits, vegetables, lean proteins and spices that are high in nutrients and don't eat white sugar, white salt, white potatoes white flour, soy milk and white rice.

Low FODMAP Diet

This diet was developed by scientists from Monash University and is a very good diet for those with irritable bowel syndrome (IBS). I have a friend who follows this diet and her body looks incredibly fit and she feels much after she started it.

Shortly, the diet consists of:

<u>Avoid</u>: apples, mango, watermelon, pears, apricots, avocados, cherries, blackberries, peaches, plums and nectarines.

<u>Eat</u>: blueberries, bananas, cantaloupe, cranberries, grapes, grapefruit, kiwi, pineapple, lemons, strawberries, oranges and mandarins.

Eat only one fruit per meal.

Avoid: beet, Brussel sprouts, garlic, legumes, artichokes, asparagus, cabbage, sugar snap peas, onions, okra, avocado, cauliflower, and mushrooms.

Eat: beans, bok choy, broccoli, alfalfa, bamboo shoots, carrots, celery, cucumbers, ginger, lettuce, olives, eggplant, parsley, potato, pumpkin, spinach, sweet potato, tomato, turnip, zucchini and yams.

Onion is the worst for IBS. Avoid it at any rate.

Avoid: bread, pasta, cereals, cakes and pastry.

Eat: rice, corn, potatoes, buckwheat and millet.

CHAPTER IX – HOW TO GET RID OF THE TOXINS IN YOUR BODY

DETOX. DETOXING IS AS IMPORTANT AS NUTRITION

Your body is created infinitely wise, by design and is programmed to be healthy.

Keeping your cells and body young depends on eating proper foods, but is just as much dependent on eliminating the toxins inside your body and keeping your digestive system healthy.

If you want to reverse aging, you have to be healthy and in order to be healthy - you have to get rid regularly of all the harmful substances and toxins your body accumulates. You have to detoxify your liver if you want your skin to look great.

Foods That Will Detox You Naturally

We have approximately 5.5 pounds (2.5 kilos) of toxic substances in our bodies, which we need to throw out.

The foods that can trigger the cleaning of the toxins in your liver and detoxify it are: grapefruit and other citrus fruits (contain glutathione, vitamin C and anti-oxidants), beets (rich in beta-carotene and flavonoids), turmeric, carrots (rich in glutathione), cabbage, avocados, garlic (contains sulphur and selenium), dandelion, apples (rich in pectin), leafy greens (rich in chlorophylls, which absorbs environmental toxins), spinach (contains glutathione), tomatoes (contain glutathione), broccoli, asparagus, green tea (full of antioxidants), cold pressed organic olive oil, hemp oil, flaxseed oil, watercress and walnuts (contain omega-3, glutathione and arginine).

CHAPTER X – THIS IS SO SIMPLE TO DO, AND PEOPLE WHO TRIED IT SAY IT MADE THEM LOOK 10 YEARS YOUNGER IN 30 DAYS

Therapy 9: DRINK APPROXIMATELY 0.8 GALLONS (3 LITERS) WATER A DAY OR AS MUCH AS YOU CAN. IT CAN TAKE 10 YEARS OFF YOUR FACE

Dehydration leads to damaging of blood cells and atherosclerosis.

The best water you can drink is the one that has been filtered by reverse osmosis or light water (I will tell you about it later on). Next comes the spring water. Some practitioners like Paul Bragg recommend distilled water and boiled water. Others say that distilled water is no good for you because it's dead and has no energy.

Mineral water provides minerals, but not in a form that your body can utilize. If you drink mineral water, try to change the types of water you drink, otherwise your body will get congested with the same minerals.

I am giving you the opinions of different experts and since they are controversial, you should drink whichever water makes you feel good about drinking it and makes your body feel good.

It is no good to drink tap water, because it is full of fluoride, which is very harmful.

Some people believe that water that comes from tops of mountains lacks in oxygen, but many people who lived longer than 100 years drank such water and it worked well for them.

You should be drinking around 0.8 gallons (3 liters) of water a day in order for your body to function properly, your cells to regenerate easily and for your skin to look 10 years younger.

If you have headaches – they could be due to dehydration.

Try this for a month and you will see the huge difference in the way you look and feel.

All organs in your body function properly when you drink a lot of water. Water flushes the toxins out of your organs and carries the nutrients to all the body cells. Your kidneys, as well as the whole of your body will be grateful to you.

Drinking more water will improve your flexibility as well – water helps to lubricate your joints.

Usually, when you have a headache the morning after drinking, it's mainly due to dehydration because your organs which need water and don't get enough, take the water from your brain and it results in a headache.

Once you start drinking more water, your complexion will improve drastically – your skin will look plumper, clearer, your wrinkles and dark circles around your eyes will get less noticeable or will even disappear.

Water can make your stomach more flat and your cellulite disappear.

It will be much easier for you to focus, since 73% of your brain is made of water and if you don't drink enough water – it can't function properly.

Drinking a lot of water will also help you eat less, because you will feel fuller without eating all that food.

Start your day with a glass of warm water with lemon and don't drink water 1.5 hours before you go to bed because you might wake up with your eyelids puffed.

CHAPTER XI - LEARN HOW FORMER COMMUNIST LEADERS WERE REJUVENATED AND HOW THEIR LIVES WERE PROLONGED ONCE THEY GOT SICK. THIS CAN PROLONG YOUR LIFE BY DECADES. YOU CAN DO IT YOURSELF

Therapy 10: LIGHT WATER

Professor Genadi Dimitrievich Berdishev is a Doctor of biology, a Doctor of medicine and was the Chief Gerontologist, who advised Former Soviet Union Leader Leonid Brezhnev, Indira Gandhi, Kim Ir Sen and Deng Xiaoping.

He shares that back in the times of the Soviet Union, a special type of water has been brought from 100 meters below the ice in Antarctica for Leonid Brezhnev, called "light water". His life was prolonged by a few years thanks to the special properties of that water. He drank such water and his food was cooked with it.

Professor Berdishev believes that human life can be prolonged by 50% with such water and he prepares "light water" for himself. You can do this as well.

Here is how it's done:

Professor Berdishev freezes in the fridge regular filtered water and then takes it out of the fridge. Once it starts unfreezing and a piece of ice as large as an egg is left – he throws away that piece of ice, which contains all the harmful elements of the water and the "heavy water" and what is left is light water. That is the water he drinks and that is that water you should drink.

CHAPTER XII – THE "GIFT FROM GOD", FOUND NEAR VOLCANOES CAN REVERSE AGING AND PROLONG YOUR LIFE

Therapy 11: ZEOLITE

According to Professor Genadi Berdishev, another strategy for reversing aging and extending lifespan is the mineral zeolite, which is naturally formed as an alchemical "gift from god" and forms where ash layers and volcanic rocks react with alkaline groundwater. Zeolite contains 73 microelements – more than any other stone. It is available on the market in liquid form, in the form of powder or dissolving tablets, so you can pick which one you want to buy. The microelements of zeolite can absorb many toxic elements from your body as a sponge.

CHAPTER XIII - REVERSE THE DAMAGE OF YOUR BODY AT CELLULAR LEVEL. HELP YOUR BODY OPTIMIZE THE FUNCTION OF THE MITOCHONDRIA AND CREATE NEW MITOCHONDRIA

There are factors on micro-level (our cells) which also accelerate aging and they are programmed in our cells. Scientists have now proven we can reverse aging at organ and system levels.

Add these substances to your diet and you will see the difference.

Therapy 12: CoQ10 Ubiquinol

Optimizes the function of the mitochondria and protects them from free radical damage. It donates its own electrons to the free radicals which are generated during cell energy production and neutralizes them.

Ubiquinol is called coenzyme because it can remain at steady levels even when it takes part in a chemical reaction.

Your body produces CoQ10 in order to protect the mitochondrial DNA, but with the age, those levels decline.

When the mitochondrial aging is in its early stages, it could still be reversed.

SHILAJIT

Shilajit is found in Tibet and Himalaya and is rich in trace minerals, Vitamins A, B Complex and P, nickel, cobalt, zink, chrome, iron, magnesium and fulvic acid. It can revitalize and stabilize CoQ10 in its active form (Ubiquinol). It also boosts the levels of CoQ10 and protects mitochondria from oxidative damage and aging.

In lab experiments, mice when given a combination of shilajit and CoQ10, have been found to have 27% more energy in their muscle cells and 40% more energy in their brain cells than when they were given CoQ10 by itself.

Therapy 13: PQQ is a coenzyme that was proven to trigger the formation of new mitochondria, protect against oxidative damage and promote nerve cell growth. A research made in 2012 was able to show that coenzyme pyrroloquinoline quinone (or PQQ) activates the genes that induce the spontaneous formation of new mitochondria in the aging cells.

PQQ was proven to be 5000 times more effective than Vitamin C at reducing oxidation.

PQQ also blocks the creation of abnormal proteins in your body.

When CoQ10 and PQQ are taken together, they can protect the mitochondria against damage and create new mitochondria. Shilajit prolongs the anti-oxidative action of CoQ10 and makes the process even more effective.

Your body doesn't produce enough PQQ and supplements are necessary.

Studies show that supplements of 20 mg/day of PQQ plus 300 mg/day CoQ10 improve the cognitive function in adults significantly.

PQQ is way more effective in terms of its mitochondria protective properties than resveratrol, quercetin and hydroxytyrosol.

Therapy 14: ANOTHER SUPER POWERFUL NATURAL ANTIOXIDANT – HYDROXYTYROSOL

A new antioxidant, which is primary found in olives and extra virgin olive oil was discovered back in 2002 called hydroxytyrosol with Oxygen Radical Absorbance Capacity (ORAC) of 68,576 is 3 times higher than CoQ10. This newly discovered antioxidant has anti-inflammatory, cholesterol-lowering, antibacterial and antioxidant effects. This antioxidant was found to improve eye health, improve symptoms of osteoporosis and heart disease. It is also able to absorb free radicals throughout the central nervous system since it is able to cross the blood-brain barrier.

Therapy 15: PYCNOGENOL

Pycnogenol is a plant extract from French Maritime pine tree and it reduces the collagen degradation and rejuvenates our skin elasticity. It also lowers the levels of blood glucose and normalizes blood pressure.

Pycnogenol contains bioflavonoids and affects the mechanisms of aging.

Studies show that it is able to improve the skin elasticity by 9% (after 6 weeks) and reduce the skin roughness by 6%, improve the production of blood cells from their bone marrow, the cellular function and the immune system in lab animals and in general, it was able to rejuvenate the animals in a better way than any other nutrient or drug.

It was also able to neutralize the damaging effects of UV light and to protect the skin proteins which break down by the UV-induced inflammatory process from degradation.

Studies on humans show that pycnogenol increases the skin hydration by 8% in 6 weeks, increases the elasticity and decreases the skin pigmentation significantly.

Therapy 16: - A NEW ANTI-OXIDANT DISCOVERED- MITO Q

A new study has been conducted by the University of Colorado at Boulder – the scientists gave old mice the equivalent of humans 70-80 years old water, containing Mito Q anti-oxidant for 4 weeks, their arteries started functioning as well as of a human 25-35 years old and they looked like young mice again. This anti-oxidant targets the mitochondria.

Researchers believe MitoQ affects a thin layer of cells that line our blood vessels called "endothelium". As people age, these cells function less properly and are less able to trigger dilation.

Past studies have shown that taking anti-oxidant supplements doesn't really help improving the vascular function in humans. This specific anti-oxidant targets the mitochondria.

When we take regular antioxidants, they don't really get to the places where we want them to go – in the mitochondria, while this new anti-oxidant will track right there.

Therapy 17 – RESVERATROL

If you eat less and exercise, an anti-aging gene in your body called SIRT 1 will be turned on.

Starving is not for everyone. Scientists have been trying to find out what would trick the body into thinking that it is getting less calories.

SIRT 1 is charged with repairing DNA and it suppresses certain genes.

Everyone has heard today that resveratrol is very good anti-aging pill, but you never quite know what is inside a pill you take, so if you can take your resveratrol from natural foods like grape seeds and skins, peanuts, mulberries and raspberries. Don't try to get it from red wine, which is a neurotoxin. It will take a few bottles of red wine to achieve the effect.

Scientists working with Dr. David Sinclaire discovered that resveratrol activates an enzyme in our body called

SIRT1, which protects us from aging. It is way more powerful than an anti-oxidant and it turns the body's genetic defence mechanisms against diseases and aging.

However, now they are already working on molecules, which are 1000 times more effective than resveratrol in terms of influencing SIRT1.

Therapy 18: JAPANESE STUDIES ON MITOCHONDRIA AND GLYCINE SUPPLEMENTS

It has been thought for a long time that aging is due to defects that happen in the mitochondria. Since it is the "powerhouse of the cell", scientists associated aging with the theory of the mitchohondrial aging or the accumulation of mutations in the DNA.

Researchers from the University of Tsukuba have recently conducted a study, which shows that this may not be the case. The study suggests that those defects might not be due to mutations in the DNA but they may be caused by external factors.

The team compared the function level of the mitochondria of children and old people and the results were astonishing: even though the older cells had reduced cellular respiration, they did not have more DNA damage than the young ones and there were no differences in the number of mitochondrial DNA mutations between both groups. The team believes that the reduced cellular function is due to epigenetic regulation, which can be reversed by reprogramming the cells to an embryonic stem cell-like state.

The scientists believe that probably the addition of certain proteins to the mitochondrial DNA might be creating the defects, which cause the signs of aging and if they "reset" the cell lines to stem cells, it would correct and remove the aging factors and that would turn an old cell to a young cell again.

The team believes that aging doesn't happen because of a damage in the mitochondrial DNA, but because genes get turned on/off over time.

They made an experiment where they restored the cellular respiration of a 97 year old cell line **after adding of glycine for 10 days and it was able to restore the mitochondria's ability to produce energy and some of the age related defects have been reversed**.

So **Glycine supplements** might become another anti-aging hit if this theory holds.

Therapy 19: TAKE LIPOSOMAL VITAMIN C – THIS FORM OF VITAMIN C IMPROVES THE ABSORPTION RATE

This form of Vitamin C is easier for the body to absorb. Liposomes are tiny vehicles for carrying nutrients throughout the body.

The liposomal Vitamin C can pass through the digestive barrier and deliver Vitamin C directly into your blood. So its absorption rate is extremely high, unlike the regular forms of Vitamin C. It might be an option to the IV Vitamin C.

Therapy 20: DHEA IS THE HORMONE OF YOUTH

Once you turn 20, your DHEA starts going down. So use a facial serum or cream with DHEA. There is not much evidence yet on the effects of DHEA taken internally, though it is known to have good effect on your skin. Dr. Perricone believes it plays an important role in your skin look.

MAKE SURE YOU GET ENOUGH VITAMIN B12

Your skin needs Vitamin B12 to look good. B12 deficiency is one of the main reasons for aging. Eat beef liver if you want to get it in a natural way.

Therapy 21: EAT WHAT RESIDENTS OF BAMA YAO WHO LIVE OVER 100 YEARS EAT – HEMPSEED

There is a village in China – Bama Yao, where population has a longer lifespan and people are healthier in general than anywhere else around the world. Researchers believe it is due to their diet, which consists of large quantities of Hemp seed, which is rich in Omega 3 and 6 fatty acids, plant based protein, vitamins, calcium, iron and fiber.

They also eat less fat and animal proteins and use less sugar and salt when cooking than we usually do in the US.

The air and the water in that village are also very clean.

The life expectancy in this village is well over 100 years. Other places similar to this are Okinawa in Japan, Sardinia in Italy and Nicoya Peninsula in Costa Rica. In all these places locals eat a plant-based diet, do moderate exercise activities and have a sense of purpose.

Therapy 22: TAKE A QUARTER OF A TEA SPOON OF ALOE DAILY TO REVERSE SIGNS OF AGING AND GET RID OF WRINKLES

A study has been conducted in 2009 – 2 different doses of aloe vera gel have been given to women at the age of 45 for 90 days – one group took a quarter of tea spoon and the other group took a little bit less than a whole teaspoon a day, and the results were astonishing: the facial wrinkles were improved significantly at both groups and the facial elasticity improved significantly at the group that was taking a quarter of a tea spoon of aloe vera gel.

So take a quarter of tea spoon of this supplement a day and enjoy the results.

Other Antiaging Supplements are:

Biotin and Sulphur - your skin needs them in order to look young and fresh;

Astaxanthin - found in algae and very beneficial for your brain;

Pterostilbene - found in blueberries, grape leaves, almonds and vines;

Cycloastragenol - telomerase activator;

Astragaloside IV - telomerase activator;

L-Carnosine - antiaging.

CHAPTER XV - THE SCIENTIST WHO INVENTED A NEW AGE-DEFYING PILL AND THE FIRST MODIFICATION IS AVAILABLE ON THE MARKET

Therapy 23: VLADIMIR SKULACHOV INVENTS AGE-DEFYING ANI-OXIDANT PILL

According to professor Skulachov, 99% of the time oxygen turns into harmless water. But 1% of the time – it turns into super oxide, that later turns into poisonous elements.

A new class of molecules, **SkQ** was synthetized by the team of professor Vladimir Skulachev in Moscow State University in 2004. It is able to deliver an extremely active antioxidant – plastoquinone into the mitochondria, which can protect it from oxidative stress.

The drug has been tested on lab rats and the results have been outstanding – the mice lived as twice as long. The professor has also tested the drug on his cataract and it has disappeared after he dropped the medicine in his eyes for 8 months.

The drug which is in the form of eye drops is called **"Vizomitin"** and can be purchased in pharmacies in Russia as well as online.

Mitochondria supplies the cells with energy. It is full of electricity.

The team of Skulachev is now working on creating different pharmaceutical products, which will be anti-aging pills. Prof. Skulachov says that the new medicine is not more complicated than penicillin and will be accessible to anyone. He believes that our life span is programmed in our bodies.

CHAPTER XVI - HUMAN PLACENTA AT AN AFFORDABLE PRICE. THIS IS WHERE YOU CAN GET IT

Therapy 24: JAPAN BIO PRODUCTS - JBP HUMAN PLACENTAL EXTRACT

A accompany, named Japan Bio Products (JBP) manufactures and cells extracts of human placental products – the placental injection **Lannaec**, placental pills and cosmetics. They use unique technologies for extracting of growth factors and other active substances from human placenta.

JBP products are not allowed for export in USA and Europe because of the existing legislation, which makes human bio products illegal on both continents. So if you want to try this product, you should go to Japan in order to do so.

CHAPTER XVII - AN EASTERN EUROPEAN PROFESSOR CAME UP WITH A SUBSTANCE THAT ACTIVATES TELOMERASE AND CAN EXTEND TELOMERES 2.5 TIMES. HE HAS BEEN USING IT FOR 15 YEARS NOW AND HE LOOKS MUCH YOUNGER THAN HIS CALENDAR AGE

Therapy 25: PEPTIDES OF PROFESSOR VLADIMIR KHAVINSON

Professor Vladimir Khavinson was nominated for a Nobel Prize for the peptides he created, which are said to extend life to 110-120 years. The Professor is now 64 and looks very young for his age. He has been taking the peptides he manufactures for 15 years now.

Vladimir says he created this medicine for his mom, who is in her 90's and who had problems with her vision, which normalized once she started taking the peptides.

Professor Khavinson claims that his peptides are able to activate telomerase and extend telomeres by 2.5 times and his team created these peptides back in 2003.

Vladimir Khavinson used to work in Leningrad Medical Academy and he developed drugs which improve the health condition of the Russian Army. That's how they discovered these peptides first. The peptides are said to be able to recover your vision within a record period of time – 2 weeks.

The Russian scientists accidentally discovered that these peptides can extend the life of laboratory mice and their lifespan was extended by 2-3 years. Same happened with experiments on monkeys.

Testing on people showed the volunteers lived 40% longer than the ones who didn't take the peptides.

Endoluten is the strongest of the peptides, which they say is able to extend lifespan. It increases the concentration of melatonin in the body.

Peptides as you know are widely used in cosmetics (face creams & serums) as well.

The products can be purchased online, but they are not cheap. The 10 –day course is sold for $ 85.

CHAPTER XVIII - HOW TO LENGTHEN YOUR TELOMERES NATURALLY AND DOES THAT MAKE YOU YOUNGER OR NOT?

Studies on prostate cancer patients show that their telomerase got boosted by following a plant-based whole grain diet and consuming very little sugar and fat within a period of 3 months. They also exercised for 30 minutes a day, practiced yoga or meditation for an hour and took fish oil supplements.

Telomeres are the protective caps on the ends of chromosomes. They are a combination of DNA and protein. As we know, telomeres get shorter and shorter with each division. Without their protective caps (telomeres), the chromosomes would just fall apart. So eventually, once they get too short – the cells die.

Bill Andrews and Michael Fossel are one of the scientists working on telomere lengthening.

Research shows that longer telomeres means longer and healthier life.

There was a study conducted by scientists at the UC San Francisco and the Preventive Medicine Research Institute, which shows that the following changes to your lifestyle can lengthen your telomeres:

Diet;

Exercise 30 mins a day 6 times a week;

Stress Management – breathing, meditation, stretching and yoga for 60 minutes a day;

Social Support

This means that people can change the length of their telomeres through changing how they live.

A study of 2014 made on African grey parrots shows that people who have high levels of social stress and are isolated from society have shorter telomeres.

A study has been made within a 5 year period with 35 men with prostate cancer as all of them were monitored closely. Ten of them made changes including plant-based diet, exercise, stress reduction and group support. Those ten men were afterwards compared to the ones who didn't make any changes and it turned out their telomeres increased in length by approximately 10%. The group who didn't change their life style had 3% shorter telomeres in the end of the 5 year period. They have checked the telomeres of the patients' blood.

Another study was done within a 3 month period of time and the participants had significantly increased their telomeres.

Scientists from Stanford Medical Center have managed to extend the length of human telomeres.

Researchers created a bioengineered version of messenger RNA that contained a coding sequence TERT (active component of telomerase) which encodes a telomere extending protein to cells.

The treated cells could divide up to 40 more times and acted much younger than the untreated ones. The team has managed to lengthen human telomeres by 1000 nucleotides or 10% increase.

The above technique is currently being tested on stem cells.

However, the effect was temporary – 48 hours after the trial, the telomeres returned back to normal.

TELOMERASE

As you know, you can slow down the cell loss by promoting telomerase. In 2011 experiments were made with mice – first they were engineered to lack the enzyme telomerase and they all aged prematurely. However, once the enzyme was replaced and the mice got it back – they all reversed their signs of aging. Telomerase can definitely reverse aging. The problem is that it can also cause cancer by speeding up the growth of the cancerous cells which exist in our bodies.

In general, boosting of telomerase also helps disease prevention.

According to Dr. Dean Ornish, if you change your diet to a whole food plant-based diet and exercise, you can significantly boost your telomerase activity in only 3 months! A group of people who changed their diets and started exercising have been checked again in 5 years and their telomeres did grow opposite to a group that didn't make any changes in their lifestyle – their telomeres have shrunk with age.

According to biologist Aubrey de Grey though, the telomere shortening is not the main reason for aging. It's only a small part of the whole puzzle.

THERAPY 26: TA-65 TELOMERASE ACTIVATOR

Most of you, I am sure know this product. TA-65 is a very good telomerase activator substance, based on Astragalus extract.

I know Noel Patton, the owner of T. A. Sciences, the company which manufactures the product. Noel is a very pleasant person, who has gone a long way developing this product. I know people who take it and they all love it - they all say they have very good results from it. Bill Andrews, who developed Product B, about which I will tell you shortly, also takes TA-65.

There was a lawsuit against the company by someone, who claimed he got cancer from the product. I tend to believe he would have gotten cancer anyway with or without TA 65. The case was resolved in favor of T. A. Sciences and the man was not entitled to damages from T. A. Sciences.

A couple of years ago, the company came up with a cream based on Astragalus extract as well.

Unfortunately, not everyone can afford TA because the monthly supply of the pills costs around $ 100 - $200 (depending on what dose you want to take) and the cream costs around $ 400.

Therapy 27: PRODUCT B

This product is a blend of botanicals and complex vitamins, created by the team of Bill Andres from Sierra Sciences. The substances have been tested and found to be able to extend telomeres. They have been adding new substances and now they have a 4th generation product on the market.

Here are the ingredients:

Vitamin A Vitamin C Vitamin E Vitamin B12 Proprietary Blend, green tea, flax seed oil, pomegranate, Milk thistle, seed extract, turmeric root extract, giant knotweed root extract, horny goat weed, herb top extract, fruit extract, ashwagandha root extract, grape seed extract, boswellia gum resin extract, blueberry fruit extract, N-acetyl-L-cysteine, bilberry fruit extract, R-alpha lipoic acid, shilajit extract, L-glutathione, Asian ginseng root extract, bacopa whole plant extract, raspberry fruit extract, canola lecithin, harada fruit extract, velvet bean seed extract, maca root extract, goldthread root extract, acacia-thorn mimosa bark extract, black tea leaf extract, white tea leaf extract, proprietary carotenoid blend (lutein, lycopene, zeaxanthin, alpha carotene), quercetin dehydrate.

Meditation

Meditation can increase telomerase activity according to a study of the University of California.

CHAPTER XIX – THE GENE THERAPIES WHICH ARE ALREADY TRIED ON HUMANS

Therapy 28: GENE THERAPY. CHANGE YOUR GENES

Researchers found out that our cells have been programmed to kill themselves. However, sometimes there are some unexpected changes that happen to human DNA and there are people who can break this program and live much longer.

There are people who lived in hell during World War II. The stress of what happened back then has changed their genes to such extend, that they were able to live to 100 easily. We have genes that can beat stress, high temperatures, etc. They can unlock mechanisms of regeneration and switch off the genes of aging. As of now there have been discovered over 3,000 genes which are associated with aging.

Gene therapy has been used on mice for many years now but it just stared being tried on people within the last few years.

Liz Parrish, 45 the CEO of Bio Viva has experimented on herself 2 of the therapies her company plans to offer in the future – one to protect against loss of muscle mass, which everyone experiences with aging and the other one to battle stem cell depletion which is responsible for aging. She was injected on September 15, 2015 at a clinic (kept in secret) in South America with a virus, used to shuttle DNA into her cells which was the carrier of telomerase gene therapy and a gene encoding the follistatin protein for people with muscle disorders, which will help her gain muscle mass easier.

Liz's telomere length was tested before the therapy and the results showed that her telomeres were unusually short for her age, which made her vulnerable to diseases. In March 2016 or 6 months after the therapy, her telomeres have lengthened by approximately 20 years – they went from 6.71kb to 7.33 kb. This means that her white blood cells have rejuvenated and become younger.

This doesn't mean though that she looks 20 years younger after she was administered the therapy. She looked much younger for her age before the therapy, so you can't see any visible difference in her look after the therapy. She looks the same, but she says she feels better and she sleeps 10 hours a night.

This therapy will be widely available for everyone who can afford it in a few years.

Therapy 29: NICOTINAMIDE ADENINE DINUCLEOTIDE (NAD)

In 2013 Harvard scientists lead by Dr. David Sinclair discovered the cause of aging and were able to reverse it and make a 2 year old mouse look and act as a 6 month old mouse by injecting **NAD +** into the 2 year old mouse. It only took a week for the change to happen. According to Dr. Sinclair, it is like a 60 year old human being turned into a 20 year old.

By administering a molecule, naturally produced by the human body, scientists were able to reverse the metabolism of a 60 year old mouse to the metabolism of a 20 year old.

Geneticist Dr. David Sinclair, who is a Professor of Genetics at Harvard Medical School has identified a chemical that may be able to reverse aging.

Nicotinamide Adenine Dinucleotide (NAD) enables the transfer of energy from food to human cells. NAD helps our cells communicate better and perform their essential functions. It gives us and our cells energy – both physical and mental.

NAD repairs our DNA, optimizes our metabolism, enhances the efficiency of Mitochondria, promotes Sirtuin Gene activation (using SIRT1 and SIRT3) and reverses the effects of aging in the brain.

We are born with high levels of NAD and as we age the NAD levels decrease and our cells can't function as properly and can't process the energy they need. Once our bodies start lacking NAD, we start storing fat, losing muscle mass, lacking energy, etc.

There are NAD supplements on the market, but most of them contain only 100 mg NAD, while you need a minimum of 1000 mg for any benefits and noticeable difference to happen. The compound is supposed to cause a similar effect to the body as if it is short on calories.

The NAD that has been used in the lab experiments was at the cost of approximately $ 1000 per drop (a daily dose for a mouse).

According to the Food and Nutrition Board, the daily doses of intake of NAD should be between 14 to max. 35 mg. However, it is always exceeded when taken for certain conditions.

NAD levels also go up naturally when we exercise or diet.

But when we age, our body produces less and less NAD and we have to find a way to boost it up once again.

NAD is derived from vitamin B3, so you may also use a form of vitamin B that acts as a precursor to NAD + called nicotinamide riboside, which is able to increase NAD levels.

Foods High in Niacin B3:

Coffee – 39.73 mg. in 100 grams

Cereal – 30-58 mg. in 100 grams

Pork – 15 mg. in 100 grams

Peanuts – 12 mg. in 100 grams

Turkey – 11.75 mg. in 100 grams

Bacon – 11 mg in 100 grams

Organ meats – over 10 mg in 100 grams

Veal – 9.42 mg. in 100 grams

Chicken – 7.8 mg in 100 grams

Tuna – 5.8 mg in 100 grams

Mushrooms – 5 mg. in 100 grams

Kidney beans – 2 mg. in 100 grams

Asparagus – 1 mg. in 100 grams

Broccoli - 0.64 mg. in 100 grams

CHAPTER XX - A NEW EXPERIMENT AWARDED BY RUSSIAN PRESIDENT PUTIN PROMISES EXTENDING HUMAN LIFE TO 200

Therapy 30: PUTIN GIVES AN AWARD of 2.5 mln. RUBLES ($39,000) TO A SCIENTIST WHO PROMISED TO EXTEND HUMAN LIFE SPAN TO 200. TAKE FUCOXANTHIN

Her name is Elena Proshkina, she is 29 and her team has been studying the Drosophilas (fruit flies) and their similarities to humans. Since fruit flies live only 2-3 months, it is easy to get a lot of research on them, change their genes and see the results fast. Human genes and fruit fly genes are 80% the same and most genes are responsible for the same functions. So if they find out what genes are responsible for aging of fruit flies, it would be the same genes for humans.

The team was able to extend life of fruit flies by 70% by increasing the activity of the genes, which are responsible for repairing of the damaged DNA and this is the first time such method has been used in the world.

So in order to relate this to humans, there are two possibilities: first is to directly manipulate the genes and the second is to get humans take certain substances which would influence the genes.

At present the team is trying different substances which would be able to stimulate the genes, which are in charge of the DNA repair. They had very good results with **fucoxanthin** which is a brown pigment, found in most seaweeds and some other marine sources.

It is stored in fat cells and can eventually induce fat loss in a few weeks.

They believe it is absolutely possible to extend human life to 200 years.

Elena believes that in 10 years there will be methods of extending human life through gene therapy, which will be safe and effective.

There are fucoxanthin supplements you can buy anywhere on the market. Do so and see how they affect you.

CHAPTER XXI - REVERSE AGING WITH THIS ENZYME THERAPY

Therapy 31 - REDUCE INFLAMMATION WHICH CAUSES AGING WITH PROTEOLYTIC ENZYMES

Proteolytic enzymes digest protein and break it down to amino acids. They also reduce the inflammation in your body, optimize blood flow, relieve heartburn and joint pain, clean and boost your immunity system. You can buy them as a supplement, made of either animal or plant sources) or you can get them naturally from food. Papaya is a great source of the enzyme papain, which can tenderize meat.

Enzymes, unlike vitamins and minerals are used in our body over and over. You need enzymes for any chemical reaction that occurs in your body. You think, breathe and heal due to enzymes. They also regulate your immune system and energy levels. Enzymes are only present in raw foods like papaya (papain enzyme) and pineapple (bromelain enzyme). The papaya has most concentrated amount of the enzyme when it's unripe yet. The nutrients in papaya also help prevent the oxidation of cholesterol and therefore prevent it from getting stuck on the blood vessel walls and forming plaques. Bromelain in pineapple was also reported to induce remission in patients with colitis. Our body does produce proteolytic enzymes (pepsin), which is often not enough because we often load it with foods that are not natural and are processed or overcooked.

When we are stressed – we get inflammation inside our body, which leads to different diseases and which ages us. Proteolytic enzymes provide protection to our body from the inflammation.

When we lack these enzymes, we have the following symptoms: indigestion, gas, heartburn, constipation or diarrhea, gray hair, lack of energy, joint stiffness, pigment spots, memory loss and premature skin wrinkles.

Here are the foods that contain most proteolytic enzymes: all kinds of fermented foods like sauerkraut, yogurt, pineapple, papaya, ginger, kiwi, miso soup and kefir.

CHAPTER XXII - BIOIDENTICAL HORMONES THERAPY – SHOULD YOU TRY IT OR NOT?

I felt I had to mention this therapy, since it really makes difference and is one of the ways to reverse aging, but I am sure you have already read too much about it and I don't want to get you bored, so I'll let you dig into the technical details on your own and will just mention a few things shortly.

Hormones are telling your body how to age and when the levels of a certain hormone changes, your aging process changes as well. In our 30s the levels of testosterone begin diminishing or what actually happens is the amount of the free circulating testosterone decreases and we can't increase our muscle mass as fast as before.

Human Growth Hormone also decreases its levels and that affects our muscle mass and our hair starts to get gray.

Our estrogen and progesterone change their levels as well. Our melatonin levels also drop.

There is an exception to the above rule - when women are about to get into menopause, certain hormones get too high first before dropping after and this can last a few years.

Hormones are chemicals that are produced by our glands (testicles and ovaries). The good news is that it is possible to trick the body get younger by natural hormone supplementation and make the body thinking the organ that produces that hormone is still young.

The problem is that all plant-derived hormone pills are synthetized through a chemical process and they are molecularly similar, but not identical to the hormones, produced by your body the way they claim on the drug labels.

One of the hormones being used by many is Human Growth Hormone or HGH.

CHAPTER XXIII – HUMAN GROWTH HORMONE – DOES IT REALLY REVERSE AGING AND WHAT ARE THE SIDE EFFECTS?

Therapy 32: HUMAN GROWTH HORMONE (HGH)

HGH has been used for a long time now by many as some of the claims are that it reduces wrinkles, decreases body fat, increases muscle and bone strength, boosts your energy, improves your vision and makes you look and feel decades younger and certainly all these claims are irresistible – anyone who can afford it would just go for it.

The FDA has approved HGH in 1996 for "deficient" adults but its consequences on healthy humans are not yet quite clear.

Clinical studies show that low doses of the growth hormone taken by adults with growth hormone deficiency can be extremely beneficial, it's mostly based on animal studies and the opinions of doctors are mixed.

Over 250,000 Americans are using bio-engineered HGH (artificial human growth hormone).

The injections are believed to be the only effective way of administering this therapy and are very expensive ($ 800 - $ 1500/month) as well as controversial - some doctors claim that they can actually upset the natural production of HGH in human body.

Some doctors believe that it's better to boost HGH through supplements than through HGH injections.

Serovital claims to raise the body's natural levels of human growth hormone by promoting the pituitary gland (the gland which produces HGH in your body) health. If you read the reviews on Amazon you will see from "I never felt better" to "a complete waste of money" and "not what I expected – I eat more than I usually eat".

Taking HGH has been proven to build muscle, but as of now studies don't show that the newly built muscle is actually any stronger.

Side effects of HGH are water retention, high blood pressure and some people even complain their nose grew bigger.

The ones who love HGH though swear by it and say that HGH delivers everything it promises like more muscle, stronger bone and they claim pain disappears.

Raquel Welch, who looks amazing at 73 shares she used Human Growth Hormone twice and it helped her deal with stress, but when she tried it later again, it made her feel bloated and puffy, so she never got back to using it again.

The best way to increase your HGH is to do so naturally.

MAKE YOUR BODY PRODUCE HGH NATURALLY

Exercise vigorously for 5 mins and relax. When running, try to sprint for 1 minute and then walk. Repeat.

According to Dr. Daniel Pompa you should exercise for 30-60 seconds, then rest for 2-3 minutes and repeat 3-4 times.

According to Klaus Oberbeil, a good way to produce more HGH is to eat a pure protein snack (fish, meat or tofu) and drink freshly squeezed lemon juice right before going to bed. Eat nothing else together with the meat. The lemon juice will help create gastric acid and the protein will be digested fully within the first few hours you fall asleep. Amino-acids will then reach all of your cells and all your weak cells will recover. Your pituitary gland will synthetize growth hormone molecules netting together 191 amino acids with the help of Vitamin C from the lemon juice. This will activate your metabolism and can both rejuvenate you and slim you.

Therapy 33: ENHANCE YOUR BODY'S HUMAN GROWTH HORMONE WITH L-ARGININE

This supplement is an HGH enhancer or in other words it stimulates your body to produce HGH. It can boost your immune system, clean your arteries and increase your blood flow, increase your bone density, increase your ability to burn fat and increase your muscle mass.

L-Arginine contains in meat, fish, eggs, diary, seeds, nuts and legumes and there is none of it in fruits and vegetables, so if you are vegan, you need to supplement with it.

You should take it approximately 2 hours before you eat anything and especially it shouldn't be taken together with protein, because it will not be absorbed properly.

Also, you should take 10 grams half hour prior to going to bed, so then your body will release HGH once you fall asleep. Take it also before you start exercising.

Make sure your L-Arginine doesn't contain lysine or HCL, because it will mean it's not a quality product and will not do the job it's intended for.

CHAPTER XXIV – DRUGS, SCIENTIFICALLY PROVEN TO REVERSE AGING

Therapy 34: SENOLYTICS

A study, conducted by the Mayo Clinic in Rochester and Scripps Research Institute in Jupiter, Florida and published in Aging Cell Magazine has discovered a new class of drugs which are able to target and kill the cells that cause aging. The drugs are called "Senolytics" and they can destroy senescent cells. These are the cells that speed up the aging process once they stop dividing. These cells act in a similar way to cancer cells – they accumulate in tissues and secret proteins which damage the surrounding tissues and healthy cells. They don't die due to their "pro-survival networks".

Scientists have found a way to induce a self-programmed death of those cells or kill them as the biggest problem has been on how to keep the healthy cells around them unharmed by the pill.

Scientists have made experiments with mice and have targeted the senescent cells with two anti-cancer drugs – Sprycel and Quercetin (a natural supplement used as anti-inflammatory). There were no negative consequences when these drugs were used with senolytics, and the mouse models have not only extended their lifespan but have also reduced osteoporosis, boosted their endurance and improved their cardiovascular functions with a single course of treatment.

The study also used human cells and this creates a big hope for the future.

Therapy 35: RAPAMYCIN (RADOO1)

A bacteria which produces rapamycin has been discovered on Easter Island.

Rapamycin is a very promising drug, which scientists believe can improve the health of elderly and delay the aging process. Tests on seniors show they got a boost of their immune systems when they used the drug.

This very promising life extending drug was originally used to suppress the immune system for people who were receiving organ transplants. It has been recently found to be able to extend the life of worms and yeast.

It was also found to extend the life of mice by up to 14%.

Some similar compounds – "rapalogs" are found to be even more effective and another drug – "everolimus" has been created, which can keep you healthy once you get old – it improves the immune response by 20%.

The study hasn't been completed yet though, and there are some side effects like increasing the chances of getting diabetes, mouth ulcers and fatigue.

Also, a group of over 200 seniors, who were given the drug showed 20% more antibodies in response to a flu vaccine, compared to a group which took placebo instead.

Therapy 36: ALT – 711

This is one of the latest anti-aging drugs and it is able to break the AGE crosslinks, which occur when glucose attaches to a protein the way it happens in the arteries. This drug seems to be promising as a drug against ameliorate aging and is very good against heart disease. Too early to say whether it will be good in a long run, because not all of the side effects have been studied just yet.

Therapy 37: METFORMIN

Metformin has been originally created as a medicine for type 2 diabetes and has been found to extend the life of small animals by 5% and according to Nir Barzialai, Head of the Institute for Aging Research in New York, it is now ready for human trials.

The above drugs are an amazing step forward in science and are brilliant solutions for people who need them. I don't recommend taking them if you don't really need them. Take as minimum of pharmaceutical drugs as you can. All pharmaceutical drugs have side effects and unless you absolutely need a chemical pill, don't take any if possible.

CHAPTER XXV – HOW TO TRICK YOUR BODY INTO CREATING NEW STEM CELLS, WHICH WILL MAKE YOU YOUNGER

STEM CELL THERAPY STEM CELL ACTIVATION

Another study of King's College, London, Harvard University and Massachusetts General Hospital researchers found that they are able to awaken a dormant pool of stem cells with a protein called FGF2 that has the ability to stimulate cells to divide and result in muscles acting like younger muscles and repairing themselves. It is also able to create new neural connections. Since scientists attribute aging mainly to stem sell exhaustion and telomere damaging, blood infusions from younger individuals might become a key to reverse aging, but I will talk about blood transfusions later. Now let's see how you can make your body produce stem cells.

Therapy 38: STEM CELL THERAPIES IN CLINICS

Billionaire Peter Nygard who is a Bahamas resident has been using stem cell therapy on himself for years and claims it reverses the aging of his body. He has been tested by the University of Miami and the results show he has really been aging backwards since doing the therapy. Nygard has been very active on making the Bahamas a Center for stem research and Center for stem cell therapies. He is a resident of Lyford Cay himself.

The Stem Cell procedure usually costs around $ 10,000 and you can do it in New York, in China or in many other parts of the world. Doctors usually take fat cells from your belly and transform them to stem cells, and then inject it back in your blood stream. In China, your stem cells are mixed with stem cells from embryos - this is also done in other countries in Asia, but not in the US because the existing US stem cell laws don't allow it.

I know a few owners of companies, who do these procedures in New York and such who do it in Asia and in Eastern Europe. They have all been using this procedure on themselves not once but multiple times, which comes to show they really have good results out of it. I also know quite a few other people who underwent the procedure in both New York and in China and they all claim they have incredible results and feel great, but it is not something that made them look decades younger or is immediately noticeable on the outside. Yet, I know these people for over 12 years and they still look the same as when I first met them if not better.

There are certain risks associated with these procedures in general - your body might reject the foreign stem cells or they might turn eventually into cancer cells, but so far I haven't heard of anyone who has had any of those complications.

MAKE YOUR BODY PRODUCE MORE STEM CELLS NATURALLY. THIS MAY INCREASE YOUR LIFESPAN BY 15-25 YEARS

Our body has a unique way to recover our sick organs and tissues and maintain an equilibrium of health. It does it through its stem cells, which are able to find the damaged organs and to divide and produce new stem cells.

Once your body starts lacking stem cells – it starts producing them.

In order for one to regain youth, they have to stimulate the activity and the division of their stem cells.

Here is what activates the production of stem cells: fasting, breathing exercises, yoga, physical exercises. The body responds to extreme activities and lack of food and oxygen with the production of stem cells.

Therapy 39: RESTRICT YOUR CALORIES - FASTING IS PROVEN TO CREATE NEW STEM CELLS

There have been many studies done on longevity and each of them shows that when you restrict the calories you take, you increase your lifespan. The first study of this kind has been done in 1930 by Clive McCane and all the rodents, whose food supply was restricted and they didn't get as much food as they felt like eating, lived longer than the ones who ate as much as they wanted. Fasting increases life span even further – the mice which have had their calorie intake cut in half and have fasted for a day, had their lifespan TRIPLED! Why? One of the reasons is that when your body digests foods, digestion creates an oxidative stress on the body and as far as you avoid that harmful process, your body regains the ability to rejuvenate. The second reason is that starving makes your body create new stem cells.

But cutting your calories also means that you have to make sure your body gets enough of the nutrients it needs, so you have to eat better quality foods instead of larger quantities. The amount of proteins, vitamins, minerals and fatty acids you take should be enough to keep you healthy.

When scientists studied how rats react on calorie restriction – it turned out that 30% of calorie restriction gave them longer life. A study on rhesus monkeys came up with similar results – calorie restriction promotes their survival and delayed the age-associates diseases.

Scientists are now working on long-term human trials on calorie restriction.

Some recent studies reveal that the effects of calorie restriction might actually be due to protein restriction instead, and more specifically - the sulfur-containing amino acids cysteine and methionine.

When researchers restricted two amino acids - cysteine and methionine, the restriction resulted in increased production of hydrogen sulfide, which protected the animal models from damages of their tissues. Foods which contain cysteine and methionine are: meat, fish, seafood, eggs, dairy products, Brazil nuts, soybeans and spirulina.

Scientists are now working on the hypothesis that pterostilbene, which is found in blueberries, rapamycin, found on Easter Island or resveratrol, found in seeds and skins of grapes may act in a similar way of calorie restriction and increase the human life span.

Many people have tried fasting, including Andrey Levshinov, a Russian author who made a successful experiment with stem cells on himself.

Andrey tested his stem cells at the Moscow stem cell bank before he started fasting. For a week he ate mainly raw fruits and vegetables and he didn't eat any meat or foods including sugar. Then he spent a week on drinking water and eating nothing and his stem cells were tested again – the amount of his stem cells at that point was lower than before. However, in the following week when he started eating again, the amount of stem cells in his body has almost doubled and in another week of eating it almost tripled!

What lead to this phenomena is that when we starve our body, it cleans the old cells, which have no much life left anyway and it creates space for new stem cells to be produced.

So try fasting 1 or two days of the week – it will improve your brain function and will make you look and feel younger.

Therapy 40: EXERCISE AT LEAST 3 DAYS A WEEK

Exercise boosts your metabolism and maintains your muscles strong.

Some call fitness a "youth serum" and it is quite clear why.

It takes one year to get visible results of rejuvenation from exercising.

Many studies show that a regular vigorous exercise can increase the production of Human Growth Hormone (also called the fitness hormone) and the production of new stem cells. Exercise increases strength, endurance and longevity and fires up your metabolism.

Physical exercises lead to creation of lactic acid and as a reaction to that, your body releases billions of stem cells in your blood stream, depending on where your body needs them – skin, hair or internal organs. These stem cells also turn into muscles.

When you do yoga, the effect is similar, but the difference is that most of the yoga poses are created in a way, that stem cells create in your internal organs rather than in your body muscles.

Research shows that 26 weeks of resistance training changes the aging process at a genetic level. It is proven that people usually lose about 5 pounds of muscle mass every 10 years on the average and resistance training can prevent that. In a way, you train your tissues to act the way they did when you were younger.

Studies show that strength training can return the gene expression to youthful levels. In an experiment, all seniors who started doing strength training had their oxidative stress revised, had 179 genes revised to their youth levels and therefore had the aging process reversed by 10 years!

Strength training has many benefits – it prevents you from muscle loss and helps you maintain good bone mass. It creates changes at hormonal, molecular, chemical and enzymatic levels in your body and it can reverse many diseases like osteoporosis, Alzheimer's, diabetes and heart disease.

Strength training can also slow down aging and even reverse it.

High intensity interval training has proved to be the most effective type of exercise, while the aerobic exercise has been found to be the least efficient one and experiments showed it could even be counterproductive.

Since aerobic training doesn't allow your muscles to rest between movements, it engages bigger part of the muscle to get used and your muscles work harder.

Strength training builds strong connective tissues and ligaments, increases your muscle strength, improves your posture and makes you look better.

As you know, strength training is the best way to help you get rid of your excess fat. You continue burning calories for up to 72 hours after you have exercised (after-burn).

The best results you can get is if you do 3 sets of 8 to 10 repetitions with heavy weights if you want to build muscles or 10 to 12 repetitions with a medium size weight for general conditioning. If the training is effective, you should be hardly able to finish the last set or you should feel a muscle failure.

Also, if you do a slow movement for 12-15 minutes once a week, it will be much more effective and will allow your muscles to burn higher amount of fat than carbohydrate and will also achieve the same production of HGH as 20 minutes of intense exercise.

When you make repetitions till the point when you can't go further, it builds more muscle mass in a shorter period of time.

Ideally, you should pick a weigh with which you should be able to do 7-8 repetitions.

You should also allow your body to rest for at least 2 days in between sessions and each time you should exercise different groups of muscles. You should do high intensity exercises 2-3 times a week.

Also, change the exercises you do, because otherwise muscles get used to the same exercise, and with time the effect of that same exercise is not the same any longer.

A recent study showed that runners in general live longer than non-runners, so running is good, but don't overdo it. The above results must be due to the fact that runners also take better care of themselves in general.

The Spine is the weakest part of the human body, because it degenerates fastest, so taking care of your spine should be a priority.

It's never too late to start exercising, but please don't wait. Start now. The sooner you begin, the greater the results will be.

AVOID EXCESSIVE SEATING

Recent studies have proven that sitting for a long time is very harmful and shortens your life, so remember to get up from your computer and walk from time to time.

There are many studies with the same results on seating which date since 1953. The first study back then was conducted on bus drivers. It showed that people who spend their time mostly sitting are at risk to get seriously ill and their chances to get a heart attack increase.

According to scientists, over 5 million people die each year due to inactive lifestyle. That could be changed very easily – by getting up from your chair and moving around every hour or so and by exercising or being active in some way for an hour each day. The studies concluded that being active between an hour and an hour and 15 minutes prolongs a person's life span.

Sitting (together with watching TV and surfing on the internet) has also been linked to depression.

Therapy 41: DO THE 5 TIBETAN REJUVENATION RITES EVERY DAY

These rites require only 15 minutes a day and the benefits from them are huge. Tibetan lamas say they can reverse the aging process and make you decades younger.

In the beginning, start doing each one 1 to 3 repetitions and eventually you will be able to do them 21 times, which is the goal. Try to do them in the morning or in the evening. They will restore your energy.

Tibetan Rite # 1

While standing upright, extend your arms at shoulder level and spin clockwise. Keep looking in front of you and let your vision blur when you spin. Continue spinning until you feel dizzy.

Tibetan Rite # 2

Lie down on your back and put your arms next to you with your palms up. Raise your legs off the ground while keeping them straight and raise your head as your chin falls towards your chest. Inhale when you start raising your legs and exhale when you bring them down.

Tibetan Rite # 3

Kneel and keep your legs together, extend your arms and put your palms on the side of your thighs. Drop your chin down while inhaling and then raise your head and lean back while you move your hands to the back of your thighs. Your head and neck should be backward and your spine should be relaxed. Then come back forward to your original position while exhaling. Keep your eyes open.

Tibetan Rite # 4

Sit on the floor and keep your legs a little less than a shoulder width apart. Keep your arms to your sides with fingers pointed forward. Drop your head toward your chest and raise your buttocks off the ground with bent knees (yoga: table pose). Your thighs should be parallel to the ground. Let your head fall back. Return into a sitting position. Repeat 21 times.

Tibetan Rite # 5

Get down on the floor in push up position. Inhale. Come up on your toes with weight in your arms and straighten your legs (in yoga: Cobra pose) arch your back and lean your head back then go into a downward dog pose while start exhaling. Try to keep your feet flat on the ground. Repeat 21 times.

Get younger skin through exercise

A recent study shows that not only exercise can keep your skin younger, but it can also reverse skin aging in those who start exercising later in life.

With the time our skin changes and we get wrinkles and sagging skin while the layer of skin beneath the epidermis begins to thin.

Researchers at McMaster University in Ontario decided to find out whether those changes were reversible or not.

They did experiments with mice and it was clear that a regimen of exercise can reverse the signs of aging in them. If mice didn't exercise, they would get ill, gray or bald but if they had a running wheel, they would keep their brains, muscles, reproductive organs and fur much longer and their fur never turned gray.

Scientists decided to check whether exercise would affect humans the same way. So they gathered a group of volunteers aged 65 or older and biopsied skin samples from their buttock (they were trying to get skin samples from the least exposed to the sun part of the body) and examined them microscopically.

After they had an endurance training program of working out twice a week, jogging and cycling for 3 months, in the end of the period their skin has been biopsied again. The second samples looked quite different from the initial ones – their skin looked much similar to the skin of a 20-40 year old. What an extraordinary result all out of exercise!

Therapy 42: QIGONG (LIFE ENERGY CULTIVATION)

Chinese scientists have studied the benefits of qigong on the human body and they claim it can reverse age associated diseases.

Qigong (chi kung) consists of meditation, breathing and physical exercises. Practitioners of qigong use their mind to guide the qi energy inside the body. It is said to be able to enhance psychic powers as well.

Clinical studies have proven the anti-aging benefits of this method. I am sure you have all heard about qigong

CHAPTER XXVI – HOW TO CHANGE YOUR BREATHING IN ORDER TO CREATE NEW STEM CELLS AND REVERSE AGING

Therapy 43: CREATING STEM CELLS THROUGH BREATHING

Another way to create stem cells in your body is through breathing. If you hold your breath, your body will feel a hunger for oxygen. In order to survive, your body needs to provide your blood with stem cells to replace the dead ones and as a result your body regenerates.

It takes 2 years to see the results from the breathing rejuvenation method.

What is most effective in stem cell production aspect is the hold of breath after exhaling - your body starts producing stem cells 12 seconds after exhaling, after you hold your breath for 60 seconds.

Bahya Kumbhaka – check out the videos on you tube on how to do it.

It is an interesting fact that animals who breathe slowly like the turtle, elephant and crocodile live longer than the cat and the birds, who breathe fast and live shorter.

Pranayama is an ancient technique of breathing and you can find many videos on you tube describing the techniques on how to do it. Pranayama can relax you, remove stress from your brain and increase your concentration.

Kapalbhati is another breathing technique.

Some practitioners recommend a breathing exercise, which consists of inhaling through left nostril and exhaling from the right one, then inhaling from right one and exhaling from left one (you can see videos on you tube if you search for **Anulom-Vilom Pranayama**). Repeat 3 or 9 times. Do this exercise everyday while repeating the **mantra Om Namah Shivaya** and you will get a lot of Prana energy in your body and will get to live much longer. After 3 months, you will feel how this exercise cleans your nostrils and eventually all of your body. Correct breathing can clean your blood, nerve and breathing systems.

When you breathe properly, you release an energy that is blocked in your body and which as a result leads to shallow breathing. Eventually that shallow breathing causes tension and diseases. When you breathe in, you should use all of your energy to do so. When you breathe out – you should do so with no effort.

When you **breathe abdominally**, you generate **Jing energy** if you drink Jing tonic herbs before that.

Therapy 44: REBIRTHING METHOD OF LEONARD ORR Om Namah Shivaya

Leonard Orr is teaching this technique, which is based on breathing. He went to India to look for immortals, to learn something from them and to study their life styles. Orr was looking for people who were at least 300 years old. The oldest one he found he claims was 8,000 years old though such claim is impossible to prove and a bit hard for us, the mortals to believe.

So what did these immortals do that was different from what all other ordinary people do? They were all using the mantra Om Namah Shivaya, which is a powerful mantra, recited by yogis in meditation. It is associated with blissfulness, grace and divine love and which is calling upon the higher self. All immortals were also all using different breathing techniques.

I will let you dig into this on your own and decide which breathing technique you want to pursue, because there are too many out there, plus I don't know in person anyone who lived to 300 and can't guarantee which one of them works best.

CHAPTER XXVII – HOW TO TRANSFORM YOUR SEXUAL ENERGY, SO IT MAKES YOU DECADES YOUNGER

Therapy 45: TRANSFORM YOUR SEXUAL ENERGY INTO LIFE FORCE ENERGY - Tibetan Rite # 6

The purpose of this exercise is to bring energy, which is usually wasted or dispersed within your first chakra as sexual energy to your 7th chakra and throughout your body.

Each time you feel excess of sexual energy, you should stand up and let all your breath leave your lungs. During exhaling, bend forward and put your hands on your knees. Bring all the air in your lungs out and stand up again. Put your hands on your waste and push. Bring your stomach inside as much as you can and stay like that as long as you can. Then breathe through your nose and exhale through your mouth and let your hands fall next to your body. Breathe in and out a few times. Repeat 3 times. Tibetan lamas say this exercise can make you decades younger if fulfilled properly and done regularly.

Many claim that sex can make you 7 – 20 years younger

Is that just a myth or is it a reality? Daoists know that the more orgasms one experiences, the more sexual energy they have circulating in their body and the longer they remain healthy and young. During orgasm we get charged with energy from the universe and the longer we manage to keep it, the longer we remain young.

However, ejaculation deprives men from their energy and that's why they feel tired and usually fall asleep after sex. Each time a man holds his ejaculation, he gets a portion of cosmic energy and stem cells. So the more often a man makes sex without ejaculation - the more energy he will receive, the more stem cells he will create and the younger he will be. Women get cosmic energy and stem cells during orgasm. So the more orgasms a woman has – the more she rejuvenates her body. In Daoist monasteries women allegedly have sex every day and they live approximately 120 years.

Therapy 46: KAYA KALPA (TRANSFORMATION OF THE BODY) CAN REJUVENATE YOU AND MAKE YOU IMMORTAL

In Autobiography of a Yogi, Paramahansa Yogananda talks about Mahavatar Babaji, who is over 1800 years old now and who may have used Kaya Kalpa to live that long.

There are 2 different types of kaya kalpa – a longer program, which involves complete isolation and a brief one. The results of the long program include a loss and then re-growth of skin, teeth and hair.

According to different sources, there are different herbs that have been used as elixirs for rejuvenation such as: pothy-karpam, gingseng, dong kwai, wheat grass juice, amalaki fruit, pippili (long pepper), aloe, ginger, neem and winter cherry.

CHAPTER **XXIX** - ANOTHER WAY TO REVERSE AGING YOU NEVER KNEW ABOUT AND YOU CAN START IT RIGHT NOW WITHOUT EVEN LEAVING YOUR HOME

Therapy 47. RAISE THE TEMPERATURE OF YOUR BODY

When your body is in a sauna or a steam room, under the high temperatures, a gene activates which controls the synthesis of **proteins of the heat shock - shaperones**. These substances are unique – they can repair damaged proteins. Thanks to them we feel great after a hot shower.

You have to bring the temperature of your body to 100 – 104 degrees F (38-40 degrees C) in order for the process to start. In order to do so, you have to not only get in a hot shower, sauna, etc., but also drink a hot drink, because otherwise your brain, which controls the temperature of your body will not allow your body's temperature to go higher than 98.6 F (37C).

CHAPTER XXX – HOW CHANGING OF YOUR BODY TEMPERATURE CAN MAKE YOU YOUNGER

Therapy 49: LOWERING OF THE BODY TEMPERATURE CAN MAKE YOU YOUNGER

One may extend their life by 30 years by lowering the temperature of their body.

Studies conducted in Japan show that mice, whose body temperature has been reduced by half degree, have extended their life span to 12-20 percent.

When you lower the temperature of your body by 2 degrees, the time slows down and you can prolong your life.

CRYOTHERAPY

This is an antiaging therapy for lowering of your body temperature. You sit in a bath filled with liquid nitrogen, cooled to -270 degrees F.

It's like you are taking an ice bath. Extremely low temperatures have a positive effect on inflammation inside your body and some of the fans of this therapy claim that it rejuvenates their skin, helps them lose weight and makes their joints feel better.

This therapy has certain risks of frostbites and there was a case of a 24-year old Nevada woman (Chelsea Ake), who somehow got trapped in the Cryotherapy Chamber for 10 hours and froze to death back in 2015.

ENERGIZE YOUR BODY WITH COLD SHOWERS

Conditioning your brain to survive and accept discomfort can greatly impact the rest of your life.

Changing the water in your shower from hot to cold can activate your lymph system and rejuvenate you. Cold shower therapy helps your body regulate your internal temperature, strengthens your immune system, improves your mood, improves your blood circulation, increases your testosterone levels, increases your metabolic rate and helps you breathe deeper.

If you can't get yourself to take cold showers, at least, get your shower to run cold for a few seconds in the end. This will have a positive effect on your body.

CHAPTER XXXI – THE EASTERN DOCTOR, WHO CAN MAKE YOU DECADES YOUNGER THROUGH A MAGNETIC FIELD

THERAPY 50: INFLUENCING THE MAGNETIC FIELD REVERSE AGING THROUGH BIO-MAGNETIC FIELD. DR. TSZYAN KANCHZHEN, (JURY VLADIMIROVICH) IN KHABAROVSK, RUSSIA

Kanchgen Jiang, a Chinese scientists living in Russia invented an experimental apparatus with a magnetic field, called Biotron.

He invented a machine that generates high field electromagnetic field and carried out experiments where old mice were treated with the aura of animal fetuses and young plants. As a result, 68 percent of the mice improved their appetite and motility, 53% increased their life expectancy by a year and a half and 31% restored their fertility.

Then he experimented on himself and his 80 year old father. Their grey hair turned into black and many chronic diseases disappeared.

96

Kanchgen also experimented with volunteers and out of 31 patients, 29 had very positive results like improvement of sex function and rejuvenation.

His experiments prove that even without interfering with the genetic system and by only changing the aura, one can get very positive results and change the fundamental behavior of the whole body.

Electromagnetic field of brain DNA is a place where the information is recorded. Its carriers are the bio electromagnetic signals. Electromagnetic field and DNA are the genetic material as a whole and its passive part is DNA and the active – the electromagnetic field. The first holds the DNA and ensures stability of human body and the second part can change it. So if you affect a person with bioelectronics signals that contain energy and information, you can change their human DNA.

In China there is a Biotron center already and people go there when they want to rejuvenate and get younger.

There is also a Biotron Centre in Khabarovsk, Russia.

CHAPTER XXXII – HOW TO REVERSE AGING THROUGH IONS

Therapy 51: REVERSE AGING THROUGH THE CHANDELIER OF A.L. CHIZHEVSKY

Your body needs ionized air from time to time and after experiments with mice, Chizhevsky finds out that red blood cells absorb negative ions which come with air and help normalize metabolism. He constructs a chandelier, which ionizes the air. The device has sharp points through which there is a flow of electrons which are increased to 100 thousand Volts.

The device produces healing ionized air - it cleans the air, strengthens the immune system and affects beneficially the blood flow.

Chizhevski believed that the diseases in human body start when the electric charge in the cells of the body are reduced. Air ions of oxygen are able to charge the cells of the human body.

Physicist Victor Zhukov claims that commercially manufactured ionizers don't have the same effect, and has built a different version of Chizhevsky's device which he has tried on himself.

The device creates protection for the human body. When the human body is strengthened and protected with such ions, it becomes much stronger.

Victor demonstrates that after he has used the device on himself for 30 mins, he can hit his hand on a desk and there is no sign of blood flow towards the spot where he hit himself and more - he doesn't feel any pain whatsoever.

CHAPTER XXXIII - IF THESE PEOPLE LIVED LONGER THAN ANYONE ELSE HAS, AND LOOK DECADES YOUNGER THAN THEIR BIOLOGICAL AGE, IT IS A GOOD REASON FOR YOU TO DO WHAT THEY DO

Therapy 52: RECREATE PART OF THE LIVES OF THE ONES WHO ARE NOW OVER 70 YEARS OLD AND LOOK 30 YEARS YOUNGER OR THE ONES WHO ARE OVER 110 YEARS. AT LEAST IT'S PROVEN IT WORKS. TOP NATURAL ANTI-AGING STRATEGIES

Raquel Welch looks amazing today at 73. She looks decades younger

Raquel shares she stays in such amazing shape through yoga and cardio exercises for 2 hours a day 6 days a week. She does 3 whole body weight trainings a week.

Raquel eats high protein (4 ounces a meal) low carb diet. She eats a low sugar vegetable with her protein. Welch eats no more than 3 fruits a day because of the high sugar content of fruits and eats only egg whites for breakfast while discarding the egg yolks.

Raquel takes ionic form of Magnesium (absorbs better), Calcium 400 mg 3 times a day, 1000 mg Vitamin C - 3 times a day and B12, Vitamin E 400 mg/day and Selenium 400 mg/day, DHEA - 5 mg/day, Licorice root, Probiotics, Shen Min (Chinese herb to nourish hair and nails), Digestive enzymes, Black Cohosh, Green Tea Extract, Flax seed, Psyllium and Armour.

Raquel wakes up around 5 AM, eats egg whites and Bieler's broth and goes to a yoga class between 6:30 AM and 8:00 AM. Then she eats poached salmon and steamed vegetables. Later she eats veal or chicken and vegetables. In the evening she eats steamed non-starch vegetables like broccoli, celery, snow peas, spinach or asparagus.

Welch moisturizes every morning and evening and she has used botox.

Whatever she does, she should continue doing it, as she looks truly amazing.

Eat Raw Like The 74 Year Old Woman From Florida - Anette Larkin Who Looks 30 Years Younger Than Her Biological Age

It is believed that vegan style of eating can reverse diseases, lose weight and even reverse aging. Vegan diets can do miracles and work well for many people and they feel and look great.

Anette Larkin is an inspiration for many. She is a 74 year old woman, who lives in Florida and looks like she is in her 40's. She never uses any kind of medication, not even aspirin. She doesn't even take B12 supplements, which most of vegans take. Anette's mother and grand-mother both had breast cancer and died young – 47 and 36 respectively.

Anette says the key to her looks is her diet and lifestyle. Anette was first a vegetarian, but 27 years ago she decided to become a raw vegan. She grows organic fruits and vegetables in her garden, she waters them with rain water and that is what she eats.

Anette drinks distilled water and gets out of bed at 5:30 AM. She also prepares natural juices every day.

Anette reads a lot, exercises and is full of energy.

Another one who looks 30 years younger than his calendar age is Bernardo La Pallo. He is now 110 years old and very youthful for his age – he could easily pass for an 80 year old. Bernardo's dad, who passed away at 98, taught him how to eat properly and he started eating raw foods when he was 5 years old. Bernardo believes you are what you eat and he eats the following foods: Honey, Galic, Cinamon, Chocolate, Olive Oil, Organic Fruits and Vegetables. He believes the fact that he has never been sick a day in his life is due to his raw food diet.

Bernardo also keeps his colon clean. Recently he drinks alkalized ironized electron clean water and feels even better. His favorite foods are blueberries and cantaloupe. Bernardo also loves carrots, cabbage, collard greens, kale, spinach, asparagus and broccoli.

Bernardo drinks cinnamon tea and eats soups. He also soaks up cinnamon bark and boils it. He gets his proteins from beans and rice. He soaks the rice to pull up the starch.

Bernardo takes walks in the morning and enjoys fresh air.

Emma Morano is now 116 years old

She was born in 1899 and says her longevity is due to her diet and habits – **she eats 2 raw eggs a day**, goes to bed early and is single. She is not vegan or vegetarian. She eats gluten. As a child, Emma developed anemia and her doctor told her she should eat 2 eggs every day. So she has been doing so since she was a young girl.

Emma eats pasta and minced meat daily and drinks brandy from time to time. She separated from her husband long time ago and never remarried.

Maria Lucimar Pereira of the Kaxinawa tribe was 121 years old in 2011

She believes her longevity is due to the fact that she only eats natural foods from the Brazilian forest like grilled meat, fish, banana porridge and manioc (root vegetable). She does not eat sugar, salt or processed foods. Maria is healthy and she walks a lot.

She was born in 1890 and her birth certificate was approved in 1985.

One of the oldest documented people in the world who lived 122 years was Jeane Calment – a French woman. Jean never actually made anything special for her health – she even smoked cigarettes since she was 21, she drank port wine and ate a couple of pounds of sweets and chocolate a week until she was 119.

She believed she lived so long because she **never experienced stress** in her life and she laughed a lot. She was born into wealth and married wealth.

Carmelo Flores was born in Bolivia and is now 123 years old. He belongs to an Andean tribe and eats their traditional diet and mainly 3 foods, which he believes have kept him alive for so long: riverside mushrooms, quinoa grains and cocoa leaves. He eats only organic foods.

Carmelo loves eating potatoes with quinoa and avoids eating rice and noodles.

He walks a lot daily and drinks water from the snow-capped peak of Bolivia's mountain Illampu. Carmelo doesn't drink alcohol.

World's oldest documented man Mbah Gotho is 145 years old as of today

As of September, 2016, the world's oldest documented man is the Indonesian Mbah Gotho. He has been just recently discovered by journalists and his documents (recognized by the Indonesian Government) prove that he has been born on December 31, 1870. Before Before this, Jeanne Calmet was the oldest documented person, who died at 122.

Mbah believes his longevity is due to his patience. He finally began to feel his old age 3 months ago, when he started needing help to eat and to bathe.

He had 4 wives, 10 children, grandchildren and great-grandchildren and great-great-grandchildren.

Russian venture capitalist Dmitry Kaminskiy has promised $ 1 million to the person who will live to 123 before knowing of Mbah's existence, So Mbah can soon become a millionaire.

The 163-year-old Dhaqabo Ebba and 171-year-old James Olofintuyi are some of the unverified world's oldest people, who have lived so far.

Shirali Muslimov – Azerbaijan's Centenarian was said to be 168 years old.

Shirali was allegedly born in 1805 and died in 1973. He credited his longevity to his active life and hard work. His diet contained of mainly yogurt, fruits and vegetables produced by his family and fresh spring water. Shirali allegedly knew his descendants down to the 5th generation.

He was very poor, but after a story about him hit the newspapers, the Soviet Government gave him a pension, which made him feel rich and foreigners came to visit him and bring him gifts. In 1964 the government organized a big birthday party for his 156th birthday and a documentary film for him was made.

Live like Li Ching-Yuen – 256 years old

Li Ching-Yuen, a Chinese herbalist died on May 6th, 1933 when he was believed to be 256 years old. He claimed to be born in 1736 while there were records of his birth in 1677, but either way, 197 years old is way longer than any other documented person so far. No one ever knew his actual date of birth, but there are Imperial Chinese Government records from 1827, congratulating him on his 150th birthday and records in the New York Times of 1877, congratulating him on his 200th birthday. According to a New York Times Correspondent, many old men in Li's village said that their grandfathers knew him when they were boys and he was a grown man back then.

Li was an herbalist and martial artist. His diet consisted of herbs like goji berries, wild ginseng, he shou wu, gotu kola and lingzhi, along with other Chinese herbs and rice wine.

According to one of his disciples, Master Li, when at the age of 130 met an older hermit, who was over 500 years old and who taught him Baguazazhang and Quigong. Li has performed the exercises every day for 120 years.

There are legends about spiritual adepts – Taoist and yogic in China, India and Tibet who have lived thousands of years.

CHAPTER XXXIV – REVERSE AGING THROUGH YOUNGER BLOOD OR JUST USING YOUR OWN BLOOD

Therapy 53: REVERSE AGING WITH BLOOD TRANSFUSIONS FROM YOUNG PEOPLE. VAMPIRE THERAPY

History has kept for us stories of people who died after the transfusion of young blood while trying to reverse the aging of their bodies. There have been experiments made on people in Germany, England and in Russia since the 17th Century, but since the doctors had no knowledge of the coagulation factors and blood groups back then, none of these experiments has ended well and the procedure has been banned.

Blood cells are the cells from which all other cells that have specialized functions in your body are generated (as described by Mayo Clinic). This is the only cell type in the body that can generate new cell types.

Studies have been conducted with mice – young mice received blood from old mice and the opposite – old mice received blood from young ones. The brain cells of the old mice, which received blood from the young ones had a burst of brain cell growth and started making new neurons. The opposite happened to the brains of the young mice, who received blood from old mice – the birth of new neurons was stalled and they began looking old. Young blood in old mice also activated their stem cells and regenerated their muscles.

Studies conducted by Harvard Scientists suggest that a protein known as GDF 11 can make the failing hearts of aging mice look like the hearts of young mice, improve the muscle, skeletal and brain function in aging mice equivalent to humans 70 years old. This same protein is also found in humans.

Scientists have proven that the blood of a young mouse can reverse the aging of an old mouse. GDF11 is found in much higher concentration in younger mice. Once its levels were raised in an old mouse, it has improved the functioning of all its organs.

Another study by University of California, San Francisco, which did a similar research, linked the anti-aging effects to a protein called Creb (cyclic AMP response element-binding protein).

Researchers at Stanford University also conducted a similar study - they injected blood plasma from 3-month-old mice into 18-month-old mice. The memory of the older mice improved.

A new report though has some controversial observations. According to the team from Novartis Institute in Cambridge and the Center for Regenerative Medicine at Massachusetts General Hospital, it is a new protein called myostatin that is the factor for the above rejuvenation. Their tests with GDF11 didn't affect the old mice at all. Turned out myostatin is 90% identical to GDF 11. The new study claims that GDF 11 actually goes up with age instead of going down.

A different study found out another factor as well – B2M, which impairs the memories of the mice.

Scientists believe that blood infusions from a younger person should be able to reverse aging effects in an older person. In October 2014, Wyss-Coray conducted the first human trial at Stanford School of Medicine – Blood plasma from young people has been given to people with Alzheimer's disease.

With age our bodies start releasing inflammatory proteins, which cause chronic inflammation. This process accelerates aging by damaging our cells.

It is known that the levels of certain proteins in blood fall with age and by the time one gets 20 years old they drop steeply while levels of other proteins increase. Stem cells stop working properly in older people and their wounds heal slower.

These studies are going to human trials now. Stem cells shut off when we turn 25. That's why scientists are now turning to blood transfusions from people under 25. There are experiments made at present with participants paying $ 8,000 per injection.

According to Wyss – Coray, what could help rejuvenation is a blend of 10 or 20 pro-youthful factors from young blood, which have been mixed with antibodies which neutralize the effects of aging factors in old blood.

Wyss-Coray found "Alkahest" – a company, which separates plasma into its parts and combines them into a rejuvenation cocktail.

One of the enthusiasts in this field is Silicon Valley's Peter Thiel, 48. He is allegedly spending $ 40,000 per month to inject himself with blood from 18 year olds. Thiel is also taking Human Growth Hormone pills.

THERAPY 54: "VAMPIRE FACE LIFT"

Have you heard of the therapy, which has people have their own blood injected into their faces? The principle is the following: A doctor, who has been trained on this procedure, withdraws a certain amount of blood from your veins, processes it to create "platelet-rich plasma" (PRP) and then re-injects the blood plasma to your face.

The procedure gives very good results and creates a very youthful look for 2-3 months and then your face goes back to its initial look.

ACTIVATE YOUR BLOOD FLOW

Hot and spicy plants are the ones to help you activate your blood flow. Many cultures have cured different diseases with hot peppers and other spicy foods. Another good source for that is apple cider vinegar, which can improve your blood circulation.

Cold showers have a similar effect on your blood flow. When you take a cold shower, warm blood flows into the skin in order to warm up your cells and beat the cold.

CHAPTER XXXV –THOSE WITH CONVENTIONAL MEDICAL TRAINING ARE USUALLY THE LAST ONES WHO CAN ACKNOWLEDGE THIS METHOD, BUT SCIENCE AS WELL AS FACTS PROVE IT WORKS

Working on your brain can add 20 years to your life span.

The secret of eternal youth is hiding in each of us and more specifically in our brains. You have to send all the energy of your cells towards rejuvenation of your body. This is certainly not easy to do, as it requires a lot of focus and discipline.

Researchers from San Francisco Medical Academy found out that aging is not written in our genes, but in our attitude to growing old and our knowledge about the process.

Reversing aging is a psychological process. Concentrate your thoughts in achieving youth and youth will come.

And don't forget that anything that pleases the mind can heal it. Our imagination projects our physical condition.

Therapy 55: CHANGE YOUR SUBCONSCIOUS THOUGHTS AND YOUR THOUGHT PROCESS

It is now proven beyond doubt by science that your subconscious thoughts can cause molecular changes in your DNA. You are your own God for yourself. Give orders to your body what you want it to achieve and how young you want it to become.

I am sure you have heard that neuroscience has already recognized that your subconscious mind is much more powerful than your conscious mind and 95 to 99 % of our lives are ruled by our unconscious beliefs, which most people are not even aware of.

Your subconscious programs might be ruining your life and your health. It is your subconscious mind that controls your life. Unless you change your subconscious beliefs, you will never be able to overcome the blocks that sabotage you and stop you from getting what you want no matter how hard you try.

A new study, published in the Journal Psychoneuroendocrinology by author Richard Davidson, has been conducted by French and Spanish researchers. It has come to prove that mindfulness practice can create changes in your body. After 8 hours of meditation for a group of people who had experience in meditation, compared to a group of people who were engaged in other type of quiet activities at the same time, the group of the meditators showed molecular and genetic differences like reduced levels of pro-inflammatory genes or faster recovery from stressful situations.

According to Dr. Bruce Lipton, gene activity can change on a daily basis according to perception. In other words, you can change your cells by changing your thoughts.

Your mind can alter the activity of your genes by changing your perception and according to Dr. Lipton, by each gene there could be over 30,000 variations of products created. One can re-write their genetic programs that are written within the nucleus of the cell through changing their blood chemistry. "Your mind will adjust the body's biology and behavior to fit with your beliefs. If you've been told you'll die in 6 months and your mind believes it, you most likely will die in 6 months." Dr. Lipton.

The so called "nocebo" effect (opposite to placebo) is unfortunately shaping our lives.

Understand that you are not a victim of your body functions and you can control your mind and your body and the doctor is not the absolute authority who is able to have any influence on your health and youth. If the society believes that you are old once you are 50, you have 2 choices – to believe them and think you are in no control or to change your beliefs and start growing in the opposite direction – growing young. The society and our parents have programmed us with certain beliefs and we need to work on changing them.

You may do your best to think positively and say all the affirmations you want, but you do that with your conscious mind and if your subconscious mind has negative thoughts programmed, the winner will be the subconscious mind and therefore the negative outcome. You are not even aware of your subconscious beliefs.

You can only rejuvenate and reverse your youth with the power of your subconscious mind. You can become who you really want to be if you don't allow a subconscious program, which you are not aware of to sabotage you.

The physical body will obey to anything your subconscious mind tells it to do. For example, people who are mentally sick and have multiple personalities – they could be allergic to a food once they express one of their personalities and at the same time eat the same food, enjoy it and have no signs of an allergic reaction while expressing a different personality.

What you think is much more important than your lifestyle. It has been proven scientifically over and over that it is not nutrition or genetics, but your thoughts determine your health and your longevity.

Stimulate mentally all your cells to regenerate daily. Be happy. A happy person regenerates while an unhappy one grows old fast. Love yourself and the people around you.

A recent Yale study on longevity concluded that people who have positive attitude towards growing old, live 7 years longer than the rest of the population who are unhappy about it.

Higher Brain Living

This is a very interesting technique and people who try it have very positive experiences. You can see videos on you tube if you search for "Higher Brain Living".

Make Your Left And Right Brain Talk To Each Other By Crossing Your Legs And Arms

The connection between your left brain and your right brain deteriorates with the years and your brain can't function properly. To fix that, cross your legs and your arms over your body and that will help make the connection between both hemispheres of your brain stronger.

Meditate With Candles

It is best if you start meditation with lighting up 1 candle and eventually light up 12 candles, but any will do better than no candles at all. Meditation cleans your soul. During meditation the time stops and you don't age. Meditation has been practiced for over 5000 years. While meditating, imagine your body with perfect organs and imagine yourself with the perfect face and body.

Therapy 56: REVERSE AGING, GET RID OF YOUR SKIN DEFECTS AND GET YOUNGER THROUGH HYPNOSES

According to Harvard researchers when you are relaxing, genes that are conductive to getting younger are turned on and genes that are conductive to aging are turned off.

In the documentary "Placebo", Dr. Albert Meissen describes how he saw a 15 year old boy, whose arms and legs were covered with warts. He was supposed to have a surgery for transplanting skin from his breast on his hand by another Doctor – a surgeon. Dr. Albert suggested that the warts should be able to go away through hypnoses, not surgery. So on the next day, Meissen took the boy under hypnoses and suggested that he will grow new soft skin and will be cured miraculously.

In a week the boy came back to the hospital and his arms were clear of the disease. The surgeon who was supposed to operate the boy previously couldn't believe his eyes because as he knew since the very beginning, it was an incurable congenital disease the boy was born with. Meissen didn't know that fact when he decided to cure the boy through hypnoses. Later on, he tried to treat other patients the same way, but he never got any positive results, because at that time he already knew that this was an incurable disease. His mind had already limited his opportunities for the future.

You don't need to use a hypnotist doctor. You could hypnotize yourself. There are also many reverse aging hypnoses videos on you tube and you can pick one that works for you best.

MANAGE AND REDUCE STRESS IN YOUR LIFE

Stress destroys the balance in the nervous system and in general shortens your life. Almost 95% of diseases start with stress. Our cells while being under stress don't get oxygen, minerals and nutrients. They become toxic and can't regenerate.

There are controversial theories on stress and according to some studies some stress is actually good for you. But no doubt stress ages you a lot because it creates inflammation in your body and inflammation causes aging and many diseases.

However, without small short term stressful situations, you will not live long as well – sometimes your body works better under stress conditions.

CHAPTER XXXVI – YOU CAN CHANGE YOUR DNA

Therapy 57: RE-PROGRAM YOUR DNA AND REVERSE THE AGING PROCESS WITH THE POWER OF YOUR BRAIN

DNA is extremely complex and it's dangerous to play with it genetically. Results could be both positive and negative. For example, Swiss scientists made changes of the gene of a fly, which was in charge of her eyes and she got eyes grown all over her body, including on her legs.

Many studies throughout the world, including USA and Canada have concluded the same: your brain activity can change your DNA. DNA is able to self-heal and if you activate this activity, you could achieve miracles.

A Canadian study made on cancer patients found that the group of volunteers who meditated managed to preserve their telomeres the same length and increase the inflammation in their bodies. As you already know, shortened telomeres don't contribute to any disease in particular, but they are one of the causes of aging.

It was believed in the past that there is nothing you can do to change your DNA and everything that happens to your body is fully dependent on your genetic code which you got from your parents.

However, it was scientifically proven, that it's entirely up to you how your genes are expressed – your thoughts matter, the food you eat matters and the environment where you live matters as well.

The Human Genetic Project discovered that our genes operate in a different way than it was believed before and it is our attitude to our surrounding which guides our gene expression. That is not only related to humans, but to microorganisms as well. Living creatures adapt to their environment and change their genes in accordance to that environment, as certain genes can be activated while others - de-activated.

What some of us know, but still constantly forget is that our thoughts – both conscious and unconscious and our emotions can literally change our genes.

In his books "The Biology of Belief" and "Spontaneous Evolution", cellular biologist Bruce Lipton explains the above in details.

Even though modern quantum physics has proven that the immaterial world which we are not able to see is far more capable to change who we are than the material one, most of us still believe in the Newtonian physics, which believes in the mechanical (visible) realm.

Dr. Lipton explains that your cells can choose which genes from your blue print to express based on the environmental factors your membranes' receptors pick up. You can choose which genes you want switched on with your conscious thoughts, beliefs feelings (love, anger, anxiety and appreciation), emotions, intentions and perceptions. Your positive mental state can change your DNA.

It has now been shown in lab testings that DNA of stem cells can be altered with magnetic field frequencies.

One can reprogram backward the stem cells and it has been recently discovered by two scientists (who have won Nobel Prizes) hat even non-stem adult cells can be epigenetically re-programmed backward, after which that can produce cardiac, skeletal muscle, neural or other cells.

Experiments have been made with a person who held 3 DNA samples and he had to generate "heart coherence" in a state of emotional and mental harmony with a heart math technique with positive emotions, and he succeeded to unwind two of the DNA samples. Other volunteers who had low heart coherence failed to do so.

Positive emotions feed our body and enhance our energy at a DNA level and scientists call these "quantum nutrients".

You are not a victim of the genes you were born with. Your body is changing in response to your thoughts and when you think of something, your body releases neurotransmitters, which allow it to communicate with your nervous system and its other parts. Those neurotransmitters are able to control your body functions and hormones.

95 % of gene mutations are believed to be caused by environmental factors and are entirely within your control (thoughts, diet, exercise, stress, etc.).

Every thought causes neurochemical changes and has the power to transform your body and your life.

Every cell we have is replaced every 2 months on the average. Cells have receptors as each is specific to one protein or peptide. When you experience a certain emotion, each emotion releases its own neuropeptides, which can change the structure of your cells. When cells divide, the new cell produced by the division will have more receptors which will match the peptides, the mother-cell has been exposed to. So whatever feelings you have – that is the way you are programming your future cells.

Epigenetics is a new science, which explains that you are a product of what happens in your life. You are the one who switches your genes on and off.

Therapy 56: REVERSE AGING THROUGH ACUPUNCTURE. ACUPOINTS

There is a point below your knee, which if massaged can bring back your youth. Chinese call it **Zu San Li** or the **Longevity point**.

Through acupuncture you can balance the flow of energy or life force which flows through the meridians of your body.

Zu San Li point is located below your kneecap between the two bones of your lower leg (there is a small dent beneath the kneecap).

You will usually feel some kind of pain when you press that point. It controls the flow of energy to your body parts. When you stimulate it by massaging it clockwise on both legs – it will improve your metabolism and the functions of your organs and blood flow. Shortly, it will rejuvenate your body.

SLEEP BETWEEN 7 AND 9 HOURS EVERY NIGHT. PEOPLE WHO SLEEP BETTER LOOK MUCH YOUNGER AND LIVE 30% LONGER

I am not telling you something new here, but I just want to remind you: A good night's sleep is crucial to your good health.

Go to bed early and get up early. Once the sun rises, your melatonin secretion which awakes your brain is inhibited. The earlier you go to bed – the better quality sleep you get. The sleep before midnight is the most quality sleep we could get.

The best time to wake up is half an hour before sunrise – that's how you catch the energy structure of the coming day. Your brain and body will have the right energy throughout the whole day. If you wake up later – you deprive yourself of that energy. You are more likely to be depressed if you wake up at 9 AM or after.

When you go to sleep your epiphyseal gland (third eye) starts working. Sleep in a dark room because studies show that light doesn't allow the epiphyseal gland which produces melatonin to work properly. Light affects you even when your eyes are closed.

Your body produces proteins, which allow the cells in your body to repair on their own while you sleep. When you don't sleep enough, your body doesn't release enough Human Growth Hormone and your skin loses its elasticity.

The best temperature to sleep at is 62 – 64 degrees F (17 – 18) degrees Celsius.

CHAPTER XXXVIII – CAN OXYGEN MAKE YOU YOUNGER?

Therapy 57 – OXYGEN AND SLEEPING IN HYPERBARIC CHAMBERS

Your cells need oxygen to function and if they don't get enough, they get weaker.

Some people sleep in oxygen tents the way Michael Jackson did, others, like NFL Players in hyperbaric chambers.

Hyperbaric chambers have become a popular practice among NFL players and many have their own portable chambers in their homes. Hyperbaric chambers increase the amount of oxygen in the bloodstream, promote healing of injuries, reduce swelling and help fighting infections.

Some have oxygen devices or exercise with oxygen masks on their face – EWOT. This type of exercise has been used by the US Military.

But scientists say that you can't really increase the oxygen in your blood by breathing tons of it. Your blood cells are 97.3% saturated with oxygen. So even if the red blood sells are able to accept more oxygen (which they are not), 3% will not make much of a difference anyway.

If you want to allow more oxygen in your body naturally, you should improve your posture, get rid of any chronic inflammation, get hydrated regularly, eat quality foods, turn the pH of your body to alkaline (instead of acidic), get rid of the stiffness around your neck through massage or exercises and reduce the stress in your life.

CHAPTER XXXIX - MENOPAUSE CAN BE REVERSED

Therapy 58: REVERSE MENOPAUSE FOR WOMEN

Scientists in Greece discovered in 2016 how to reverse menopause. Women who haven't had their period for 5 years were able to menstruate after their ovaries were rejuvenated.

This was made possible with platelet-rich plasma (mix of substances in the blood) – RPR, that help cells grow and are able to stimulate tissue regeneration. Now post-menopausal and older women are already able to conceive. This method can also work in rejuvenation of older ovaries.

Dr. Konstantinos Sfakianoudis, a gynaecologist is leading the team of Doctors who made that possible at the Greek fertility clinic Genesis Athens.

Therapy 59: SHRINK YOUR BELLY AND YOU WILL LOOK AND FEEL DECADES YOUNGER

A flat belly can take decades off your appearance and make you look younger and more attractive.

It's great if you do abdominal exercises like crunches, but unless you combine that with the proper diet – there will not be much of a result, as your fat stores will not be affected much.

A flat belly is 80% result of good diet and 20% related to exercise, sleep and less stress.

Reduce Stress – stress causes cortisol (a hormone in your body that holds on to fat in your abs) levels to spike;

Eliminate sugar, fructose, grains which break down to sugar in your body and processed foods;

Eat good fats like salmon, avocado and walnuts;

Eat mostly raw foods;

Eat fresh vegetables;

Avoid diet foods, snacks, dried fruits and sweetened yogurts;

Slow down your breathing;

Avoid artificial sweeteners;

Eat foods rich in vitamin C;

Push-ups are very effective for the abs;

A very good exercise is also pulling your belly back towards your spine and holding while you lie down or even while you walk. Breathe while doing so;

Get enough sleep – it is important for your body to regulate your metabolism properly. Studies show that people who sleep less accumulate fat easier;

Do high intensity interval training, which is more effective than long time training 20 minutes 2-3 times a week. Studies show that you can lose more weight if you exercise intensely for a shorter period of time.

Building your abs also helps you to stabilize your spine and disks.

CHAPTER **XXXX** - LONGEVITY THERAPIES THAT HAVE BEEN PROVEN TO WORK

I will only mention these therapies as they are common-sense things to do and I have written about them in my other books, but I want to remind them to you.

Get Younger through the sun – your body needs sunlight

It is well known that Ultraviolet sunbeams make our skin older. But when our skin receives photons from the sun, it promotes our body to produce Vitamin D and the more Vitamin D our body has, the more our metabolism will increase.

The best sun is before 8 AM. Try to get at least 20 mins of sun every day.

Intellect - People with higher intellect have been proven to live longer.

Breathe fresh and clean air

Have as much joy in your life as you can

Optimism can extend your life by 8 years

Love and happiness add 15 years to your life

Be active as long as you can – mentally and physically

Think Positive. Negative thoughts and attitude age you.

Hot and cold showers (Cold-hot – change 3 times and finish with cold).

Take care of someone

Experiments show that the ones who take care of someone live longer than the ones taken care of. So make sure you are needed.

Oil pulling

I recently told a friend of mine to try whitening her teeth with coconut oil pulling and she called me 2 weeks later and told me that it changed her life – she said she looked better, felt better and slept better since she started doing it.

Proper posture

When your posture is straight – you look 15 years younger.

Express gratitude as often as you can

Create for yourself the perfect living conditions

An experiment was made, which concluded that if people live like the volunteers who took part in the experiment and who spent 3 years in perfect conditions, they would live till 165 if they lived like that till the rest of their lives.

Neuropeptides (endorphins or hormones of happiness) can prolong your life and reverse aging

Massage of your spine and a whole body massage can rejuvenate you

Get a quality brush and comb your hair every day. This will give a great massage to your head

You have to enjoy life, or else you will get sick

Wear only clothes from cotton and other natural materials

Create your personal philosophy for immortality. Every night repeat to yourself that tomorrow you will be 5 years younger. Order your cells to create new ones - stronger, younger and healthier and to replace the old ones.

Listen to music you like - it creates higher vibrations in your body

Clean your energy

If you spend time with people who are sick, dying, narcissists, sociopaths, psychopaths or energy vampires, your energy will get contaminated and you will grow old very quickly. Try to surround yourself with people with zero negativity, people who bring out the best of you and people who have good energy only.

Watch the sun at sunrise and the moon during night and you will be charged with a great amount of energy

Jump to increase blood circulation

Avoid all toxic cleaners in your home

Do your best to use organic and non-toxic soaps, dish cleaners, shampoos, sprays, etc.

LIVE IN A PYRAMID

Pyramids are unique and they can stop the time. According to scientists one has to spend 15 mins a day in a pyramid and the time will start going in the opposite direction.

LIVE IN A MONASTERY

Viktor Vostokov describes his studies in a monastery where he studied from Tibetan lamas and where he saw things that are beyond limits of human consciousness. He describes how lamas work daily and how some of them can even bring death people to life. Lamas study for 20 years and they can heal with a glance, heal with a thought or with a pray. They can diagnose your diseases by your tongue, pulse, nails, teeth, ears, aura and spine. Lamas learn how to prepare different elixirs. They can do bio-massage, phyto-therapy, relaxation, needle-therapy, etc.

Tibetan healers believe that the normal functioning of the body depends on the availability of qi energy.

Learn new things every day like this one for example:

Psychoneuroimmunology can teach you a lot about the interaction between the nervous system, the immune system and psychological processes of the human body and it studies the integration between thoughts, emotions, and physical reactions at a cellular level.

Therapy 60: FACIAL EXERCISES - GET RID OF WRINKLES NATURALLY

Facial exercises can strengthen your face and neck and will rejuvenate you.

I will let you dig on this on your own. Once you go to you tube – you will see many videos and pick the exercises that you need for your face type.

Facial exercises can make a big difference in the way you look, but it doesn't happen overnight. It takes time. You will see results 2 weeks after you begin doing them.

It does reduce wrinkles and puffiness and improves skin texture. You tighten and tone the muscles in your face.

You have to provide your skin with enough oxygen in order for it to stay healthy and that means good muscle tone and circulation.

Topically applied anti-oxidants

Topically applied antioxidants like CoQ10, Vitamins C and E rejuvenate and protect the skin.

Some scientists now believe that **coffee berry** is even a more powerful antioxidant. It was found to improve the appearance of fine lines and wrinkles.

Peptides applied topically

I introduced you to peptides taken as a pill earlier in the book, and will now mention peptides in cosmetics about which I am sure you have all heard about. Formulations like Argireline for example can produce a botox-like effect and inhibit the release of neurotransmitters which keep the facial muscles from forming wrinkles. Peptides stimulate your skin to look much like younger skin.

Therapy 61: ONE TRUTH 818 SERUM

This is a newly developed serum, which is not yet available on the market (but will soon be), which has been developed with the help of the anti-aging molecular biologist Dr. Bill Andrews of Sierra Sciences. The serum contains a Telomerase Activating Molecule TAM – 818, which has been discovered by the team of Dr. Bill Andrews.

Therapy 62: THREADING FACE LIFT

This scalpel free procedure has been discussed a lot and it's one of the procedures Gwyneth Paltrow likes. Some call it "under the radar approach" to anti-aging. The FDA didn't approve the procedure, but it is widely popular in Europe and Asia. There could be side effects from this procedure, so unless you go to a Doctor who knows what they are doing, you'd rather pass on it.

CHAPTER XXXXII - THE SECRET OF SKIN DOCTORS

Therapy 63: TRETINOIN CREAM - THE SECRET OF ALL SKIN DOCTORS

This is the secret of all Dermatologists. They all use one and the same face cream – Tretinoin (Retin A). Retinoids are derivatives of Vitamin A and they increase collagen production and decrease collagen breakdown. And most of them use the 0.1%. This cream is prescription only and the price is around $ 80 for a small tube. Certainly listen to what your Doctor says, but it's best to start with 0.025% or 0.05 % one and never use it during summer, because you may get pigmentation. Always use sunscreen while you are using it - even in the winter.

Therapy 64: MICRO-NEEDLING

Buy one of these micro-needle rollers online and roll on your face and neck once a week while using one of your favorite serums. It is not the most pleasant procedure, but it gives good results.

Vitamin D

I met Dr. Patricia Wexler – a very famous Manhattan dermatologist at an event in New York. She looks amazing and decades younger at 73. She shared that her secret for her good skin is staying out of the sun while taking vitamin D supplements to compensate for the lack of sun. She also uses Ulthera laser herself and is loving the results.

Put oil or hydration lotion on your body every day

After the age of 40, you have to start putting oil or hydrating lotion on your body every day.

Spray purified water on your face a few times a day

Rub Ice cubes on your face to get a natural healthy glow

Use on your face tonic with half apple sider vinegar half water and some lemon

Put vitamin C serum and aloe on your face

Lie down for 10 minutes with cold and wet green tea bags on your eyes to rejuvenate your eyes

Make dark circles mask out of aloe, licorice extract and vitamin K

Chemical peeling and photo peeling

The mechanism of activation of stem cells is widely used in cosmetic industry and chemical peeling is an example. When there are critical conditions created for our skin – in a moment of mass death of cells - it starts producing new stem cells.

Wash your face with aspirin

Exfoliate your face with Aspirin and you will have no black spots – wash your face with aspirin dissolved in warm water.

Brush your skin

This is how you get rid of all the dead cells and your skin releases the toxins. Brush in a direction towards your heart.

GET RID OF SKIN PIGMENTATION

Skin pigmentation – dark spots, freckles, warts, etc. can make you look 10 – 15 years older – no doubt about it.

What causes skin pigmentation?

UV exposure is certainly the number one reason for pigmentation – it increases the melanin production;

Heat – your cells which produce melanin don't react well to heat and they produce pigmentation as a result of it. Thermal radiation affects melanocytes the same way UV does;

Medications – some medications cause hyperpigmentation as a side effect;

Injuries – often after a wound heals and there is still inflammation left in the place of the wound and it creates pigmentation;

Stress
Emotional stress was also found a culprit for skin pigmentation. Even though short term stress can increase your life span, it can affect the skin production of melanin.

Hormonal Changes

Treatment of pigmentation:

All the ingredients below are known to reduce skin pigmentation. The more of them you mix together and put on your face – the better. Leave for 15 minutes or so and rinse with water.

Lemon mixed with honey will act as a natural bleach.

Lemon Juice plus Turmeric left on your skin for 10-15 mins can give good results. Make sure you don't expose your skin to sun right after using the lemon on it.

Cucumber mixed with lemon and honey, Aloe Vera (clears dark spots), Yogurt, Tomato, Red Onion (rub the sliced onion on the spots), Potatoes (can lighten your pigmented skin and dark spots – rub the sliced potato on your skin daily. They contain high amounts of catecholase - a potent skin lightening ingredient), Buttermilk, Orange peel, Apple Cider Vinegar mixed 50/50 with water, Avocados, Banana, Guava and Sandal wood powder.

Healthy balanced diet.

Use sunblock to prevent further pigmentation.

Sunscreens

Most sunscreens protect us against UVB rays. There are now two new technologies in sunscreens – Heliopex is a new technology that makes the sunscreen ingredients more effective and Mexoryl SX is a new protective agent, which defends against the aging effects of short UVA rays.

I am sure you know that you can get pigment spots even when the weather is cloudy, but I want to remind you to use sunscreen even in cloudy weather. Also, many forget to put sunscreen on their hands and that's why their hands age first.

Get rid of turkey neck or neck bands

Our skin loses elasticity with age while our neck muscles get stronger and we get neck bands or turkey neck.

Use creams with retinoids, hyaluronic acid and Matrixyl and creams that moisturize the skin well. Also good are creams with Argireline, sesaflash and shea butter.

Do facial exercises. Once you build the muscles in the chin and neck area – the skin will get smoother, firmer and will tighten.

Do facial massages, which will increase the blood circulation and will tighten the neck.

Drink a lot of water to hydrate your skin. When your body is dehydrated – it leads your neck skin to create turkey neck. So drink 8 glasses of water a day.

Limit the amount of salt you eat – sodium can cause water retention in the neck.

Massage will not improve your muscle tone like facial exercises, but can be very beneficial for your skin.

Fractional CO2 Lasers

They are being called the "antiaging breakthrough of the decade" and the procedures cost around $ 2,500 - $ 5,000. They really work and make miracles, but unless you stay away from the sun like from a plague, chances are you will get pigmentation after – it happened to anyone I know who went through it even though anyone of them used sunscreen.

Get rid of stretch marks

Use the following natural substances to rub on your skin (and leave for 15 mins before rinsing) daily for at least 30 days and get rid of stretch marks: Castor oil, Aloe Vera, Lemon Juice, Alfalfa(rich in vitamins like E and K and minerals), Cocoa Butter (moisturizes), Olive Oil (rich in antioxidants), Sugar (exfoliates).

Therapy 65: REVERSE THE COLOR OF YOUR GRAY HAIR

Gray hair is usually blamed on genes, stress and aging.

The color of the hair comes from a pigment, called melanin (it can be dark or light). The protein keratin gives our hair its color. As we age, melanin is reduced. Oxidative stress and vitamin B12 deficiency are among the other causes of gray hair. There are cases of hair returning its pigmentation after B12 deficiency is restored.

Scientists discovered that as we age, we produce less catalase enzyme, which results in aging.

DNA damage and oxidative stress can be reduced by such enzymes like catalase.

Our hair cells produce hydrogen peroxide and it starts building up in the hair and can't be broken down because of less enzyme catalase, which causes the hair to turn gray.

Supplements that increase the activity of catalase in laboratory rats have slowed down the aging process in them.

Natural source of catalase is **wheatgrass**, which has 92 minerals and 19 amino acids and has detoxifying properties. It also contains vitamins, amino acids, chlorophyll, enzymes and nutrients. Our body can absorb the nutrients from the wheatgrass fast because of the similar molecular structure with our blood cells.

Drink a glass of wheatgrass juice every day or put wheatgrass powder in your juice.

Also, apply wheatgrass juice on your scalp and leave it for 5-10 minutes before you rinse your hair.

The first gene related to gray hair has been discovered recently.

Researchers have been working to get to the root of the problem and reverse gray hair to its original condition. Scientists at the Langne Medical center of New York University have isolated a wnt protein which coordinates pigmentation and when they inhibited it in black mice – they turned gray. Researchers believe that one day they may add this protein to hair products and cure gray hair permanently.

It has also been found that a compound called **PC-KUS** could reverse and "cure" gray hair.

Scientists believe to be able to reverse gray hair from the inside soon.

Other natural ways to get rid of gray hair are to apply on your scalp and keep for 1 hour on your hair a mixture of the following ingredients (or as many of them as you have at home):

Coconut Oil, Curry Leaves, Indian Gooseberry (rich in Vitamin C and other antioxidants), Rosemary, Sage, Henna, Amaranth Juice and Black Tea.

Massage your scalp with **onion juice** and rinse after 30 mins.

Eat a spoon of **blackstrap molasses** daily for a few months. It produces a pigment, which will help your hair return its natural color and is also rich in magnesium, iron and selenium.

Also eat a teaspoon of **black sesame seeds** daily for a few months. It boosts production of melanin.

Supplements that help your hair keep its color are Vitamin B5, Folic acid, Biotin and Pantothenic acid or you should eat salmon, cod, trout, egg yolks, unprocessed rice and nuts. Your hair also needs tyrosine, so drink the juice of 1 lemon or drink a glass of apple cider vinegar mixed with water.

Therapy 66: GROW NEW TEETH AT ANY AGE

A few Russian authors as Mikhail Pillars for example have published books in Russian on how to grow new teeth even when you are in your 40s and 50s. They do it with the power of their brain the same way you can reverse aging of your whole body with the power of your mind.

A Harvard team of scientists has found a way to regrow teeth. They used a low-power laser beam and triggered human dental stem cells to encourage them to form dentin (hard bone-like tissue). Until now it has been difficult for scientists to coax the stem cells into becoming specific types like dentin for example. This new laser method is a big step – it is faster and less invasive.

SECOND SKIN

And if all the above treatments don't achieve the effect you are aiming for, there is yet another chance for you to look amazing: the newly invented "second skin".

Modal Trigger Scientists developed it for cosmetic purposes like reducing your under eye circles. It is a silicone – based polymer solution that provides an ultrathin second skin layer that smooths under eye wrinkles and tightens skin. Researchers from Harvard and MIT spent 10 years in developing it.

It also locks the moisture and can prevent UV exposure.

The effect will last approximately 24 hours. As of now, it hasn't yet been approved by the FDA.

CLEAN THE AIR IN YOUR HOME WITH PLANTS

Some plants can improve the quality of your air at home. As we know, plants convert carbon dioxide to oxygen through photosynthesis. They also can absorb harmful gases and clean the air in general and keep us young and healthy.

NASA published a study in the 80's which gave proof that plants have very positive influence on us. NASA and Associated Landscape contractors of America studied different plants indoors and their effects on humans.

Turned out some plants improve the quality of air and absorb the pollutants in the air. NASA even sent plants in space in order to keep astronauts with a good supportive environment and keep their air healthy.

Bamboo palm and all spider plants were found to remove formaldehyde in the air while daisies, mums and English ivy were able to remove benzene. Here are some plants that are the best choice for your air quality. English ivy, elephant ear philodendron, heartleaf philodendron, cornstalk dracaena, spider plant, weeping fig, golden pothos, Chinese evergreen, Janet Craig dracaena, Warneck dracaena, `Mauna Loa', peace lily, selloum philodendron, bamboo or reed palm, snake plant and red-edged dracaena.

CHAPTER XXXXIII – THIS MAN TRIED IMMORTALITY ON HIMSELF AND HE IS DOING GREAT

THERAPY 67: 3.5 MILLION-YEAR OLD BACTERIA BACILLIUS F

Bacteria have been found in the ancient permafrost in Yakutia and its DNA has been unlocked already. It has been tested on mice and on human cells.

Russian scientists lead by Dr. Anatoli Brouchkov believe that this bacteria may increase the lifespan of humans. They are trying to understand how they have survived for 3.5 million years in Siberian permafrost.

The bacteria have a positive effect on humans, mice, plants and fruit flies – they stimulate the growth of crops and strengthen the immune system.

Similar bacteria have been discovered in the brain of an extinct wooly mammoth preserved by permafrost.

The scientists don't yet know the mechanism of how they work, but the positive impact of the bacteria is obvious.

The mice grannies, on which the bacteria were tested, produced offspring. The bacteria could improve the life of humans and act as an elixir of life for the future.

If scientists manage to find out how this bacteria protect themselves from damage (something our cells are not able to), it might help scientists figure out for us how to live forever.

According to Dr. Victor Chernyavsky, the bacteria activate the immune status of experimental animals.

Anatoli Brouchkov has injected himself with the bacteria and says he feels healthy and hasn't caught flu within the last 2 years (since he injected himself).

But don't get too excited - even though Anatoli looks great for his age, he hasn't grown decades younger since administering that injection, as we all wish he did.

CHAPTER XXXXIV A NEW HORMONE REVERSES AGING

Therapy 68: A NEW HORMONE - DANAZOL FOUND TO REVERSE AGING

A synthetic male hormone **danazol** was found to reverse cell aging. As it is known, the human body can heal itself on its own but it can also regenerate dying cells.

Scientists from US and Brasil made experiments with a synthetic male hormone – a danazol steroid and tried to arouse the production of telomerase. Telomerase can stop aging and the process is similar to blood forming cells.

Danazol has been tried on patients with aplastic anemia (caused by mutation of telomerase genes).

A person with the above disease would lose from 200 to 600 telomere base pairs each year compared to 100 to 120 telomere base pairs for a regular healthy person.

However, the intake of the hormone has side effects such as fatigue, digestive system problems and mood swings. The length of the telomere cells of the patients stopped shrinking and even increased by 386 base pairs on the average. Hemoglobin mass also increased and they no longer needed to have blood transfusions.

CHAPTER XXXXV - TREATMENTS COMING UP IN THE PIPELINE WHICH SHOW AMAZING RESULTS ON ANIMAL MODELS AND ON HUMAN CELLS, BUT ARE NOT YET WIDELY USED ON HUMANS

It has been a desire of humanity to extend their life since the beginning of time. Immortality would be the greatest possible discovery and reward of human progress and it will be here soon.

Today the possibilities of new medical miracles look more doable and promising than ever before.

Futuristic projects are now cropping everywhere around the world. Anti-aging drugs have been in a development for a long time. The elixir of life or the vaccine for death will be here within a decade.

Google founded a company, focused on health and wellbeing – Calico. The Human Longevity Project, which aim is to target ageing related diseases, managed to secure $ 70 million only in the first round of financing.

Here are the most interesting and most promising discoveries so far:

FOOLING THE GENES

Back in 2011 French scientists were able to restore the youth of cells taken from a 74 years old patient and reprograming them to stem cells stage. That demonstrates that aging is in fact reversible.

Richard Dawkin describes this method of fooling the genes into thinking that the body is young again. We have genes in out body that activate at a different time throughout our life span and their activation is triggered by environmental factors. We trigger more lethal genes when we get older, so in order to extend our lifespan, we should find a way to prevent them from switching on by changing the internal chemical environment of our body to that of a young body.

CHINESE SCIENTISTS DISCOVER GENE P16 RESPONSIBLE FOR CELL AGING

Scientists from the Beijing University found out the gene, which is responsible for cell aging and they believe that the process of aging is coded in the cells. Once this gene gets blocked, the cells can reach immortality and this will become possible with the development of nano-technologies. There will be nano-robots created with the dimensions of a bio-molecule. These robots will create local electromagnetic fields, which will form chemical changes in the bio molecules. Those robots will also help the cells get rid of the harmful free radicals and they will switch on/off the corresponding genes.

NANOTECHNOLOGY

Nanotechnology will help anti-aging through repairing of the aging process with the help of cell repair machines or mini robots, which would be able to go inside our bodies and will operate within our cells.

115 YEAR OLD WOMAN'S BLOOD GIVES OUT A SECRET

Hendrikje van Andel-Schipper died in 2005 when she was 115 years old and she was in a good health almost until she died.

Scientists at the VU University in Amsterdam found 450 somatic mutations within her white blood cells, which however weren't associated with any diseases. It also turned out that the majority of her white blood cells were derived from just two stem cells (we are born with approximately 20,000 blood stem cells).

Also, the telomeres of her white blood cells were very short and around 17 times shorter than those of her brain cells.

After analyzing the above results, scientists made a conclusion that probably the reason we die is because our pool of stem cells slowly diminishes and in the end we are not able to regenerate tissues.

So probably one day it will be possible to rejuvenate the body with stem cells from the person when they were younger and that might only be possible with blood stem cells.

REVERSE AGING IN 5 YEARS THROUGH CRISPR

According to George Church, a genetics professor at Harvard Medical School, who spoke in front of the Washington Post, his team will be able to reverse aging in 5 years. It is already happening with mice in the lab.

They have been using a recently developed gene-editing tool –CRISPR to edit the mice's genetic code.

Unfortunately, it didn't work quite well with people –
only 4 out of the 54 human embryos exhibited genetic
changes.

BIOELECTRONICS MEDICINE

Google's "Verify Life Sciences" and "Glaxo Smith Kline"
started a new company – "Galvani Bioelectronics",
which is going to develop bioelectronics medicine.

The regulators of body's organs and functions are
circuits of neurons. Scientists believe that they can
implant small devices in the human body, which can
sense all irregularities and can deliver impulses to turn
diseases on/off.

Many studies recently managed to prolong life of cells in
laboratory conditions. Researchers from Korea found a
synthetic molecule - CGK733, which is able to cause a
cell divide 20 times more than it normally would or in
other words increase its life by 25%.

LACK OF GRANZYME B

While a team of researchers from the University of
British Columbia was studying blood vessel
deterioration in mice, they witnessed something
unusual - the mice that had been engineered to lack
Granzyme B had very smooth skin whereas the rest of
the mice had aged skin.

Granzyme B is produced by the immune cells and is
able to break down other proteins.

An experiment was made with exposing mice to sun for
20 weeks and in the end of the trial, the mice lacking
Granzyme B had smooth skin, while the rest of the mice
started to get their skin wrinkled. Turns out the
immunity system can cause other cells self-destruct.
For example, after sun exposure the levels of this

enzyme in your body go up and your immune system can destroy sun damaged and virus infected skin cells without even knowing.

FIBROPLASTS

Scientists from USA and Japan independently from each other discovered that if they deliver through viruses additional genes in the skin of an old person, they can re-program the cells to start producing stem cells. This results in younger skin.

WHAT MAKES THE HYDRA IMMORTAL? THE FoxO GENE MAKES HUMAN LIFE LONGER

The fresh water polyp hydra is immortal. It contains stem cells, which are capable of continuous proliferation. Many studies are being done to find out how come the hydra is full of stem cells throughout its life.

The FoxO gene has been found in the hydra, which exists in all animals and humans but until recently no one knew that it might be connected to aging. In a study carried out by Kiel University, researchers isolated the stem cells of the hydra and screened its genes and it turned out that once they switched off the FoxO gene, the hydra had very few stem cells and its immune system changed as well.

Same was found to be valid for humans. People in whom this gene was very active lived longer – more than 100 years. It is not possible to genetically manipulate humans and find out whether that hypothesis is true, but scientists are trying to find different ways to check that out.

INDY GENE INCREASES LIFESPAN AND PROLONGS FEMALE FERTILITY

Scientists from University of Connecticut Health care managed to double the lifespan of fruit flies by genetic alteration of their Indy gene. The insects also remained physically and sexually active much longer. These mutations extended their life span by creating a metabolic state similar to calories restriction. So calories are either wasted or not absorbed. The genetic alteration didn't affect their appetite, which means they could eat as much as they want and still age as twice as slower. So this gene will also help fighting obesity.

Humans have the same gene. Decreasing its activity in humans should also mean longer lifespan.

This was the second gene found to be able to prolong lifespan of fruit flies. Females also continued to produce offspring for 40% longer than average.

REVERSING AGING THROUGH ERADICATING MITOCHONDRIA

Scientists from the UK Institute for Aging at Newcastle University made experiments where they found out that once they removed the mitochondria from human cells, that process lead to rejuvenation. Some cells in our bodies lose the ability to replicate and once that happens, they build up over time and cause damage to the surrounding healthy tissues by producing oxygen species (oxidative stress).

The team grew human cells in a lab and removed almost all the mitochondria. Once the mitochondria were removed, that triggered the rejuvenation of the cells. Now the team will work on antiaging therapies which target the mitochondria.

CLEARING "CELLULAR LITTER" EXTENDS LIFE OF MICE BY 35%

Researchers from Mayo Clinic in USA found that senescent cells (cells that are growing old) that no longer divide and accumulate are one of the causes of aging and once those cells were cleared on lab animal models, the mice lived 35% longer. Since those cells secrete certain proteins, which have a negative impact on all the surrounding cells and organs, once they got cleared, the mice got rejuvenated.

Researchers genetically modified mice so they would respond to AP20187 – a compound, originally developed as an anti-cancer drug.

This compound would only be effective in humans if they took extremely large dozes, which would on other hand make it toxic, but there are now drugs being developed, which are based on this same concept of taking out cellular "trash".

And in the end, one last secret – all the above therapies you should do with enthusiasm. If you are not enthusiastic about reversing aging, there will be no results. Enthusiasm is the main driving force of your brain and body.

I recommend reading this book or at least the therapies you could do on your own every day for 40 days until it becomes a habit (it takes 40 days to form a habit) to do the things you need to do and reverse the aging process of your body and you will see results very soon after.

Reversing aging is not an easy job – it requires a lot of will, discipline, time and money. The results though will be worth it. We are first wasting our heath and youth and then are hoping to find a pill which would be able to give it back to us miraculously.

I can't promise you the results you want to achieve, because they are entirely up to you, but if other people have achieved them, you can do it as well!

According to Aubrey de Grey, it is much easier for scientists to reverse aging than to stopping aging from happening. But that doesn't mean you should wait to get old in order to start taking the pill they come up with tomorrow. Your youth is in your own hands.

Some call the quest for eternal youth "crazy" or "creepy", but I believe it's the ultimate reward.

If you are working on an antiaging project and you need financing or help to commercialize it, or if you want to invest in a project that reverses human aging, e-mail to: valnyc2005@yahoo.com

Dear Reader,

If you liked this book and it helped you in one way or another, I would really appreciate if you write a few words as a review and say what you think about it.

Thank you!

Other Books from the same Publishing House:

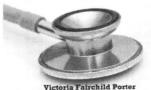

**58 Effective Cancer Therapies
Backed Up By Science
You Probably Never Heard About**

Get Rid Of Any Kind Of Cancer And
Any Other Disease Fast With No Side Effects

Plus: 47 Natural Anti-Cancer Substances

Plus: 12 Controversial/Forbidden Therapies

Victoria Fairchild Porter

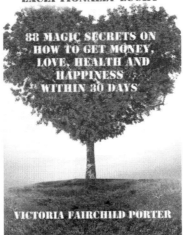

HOW TO MAKE EVERY DAY
EXCEPTIONALLY LUCKY

88 MAGIC SECRETS ON
HOW TO GET MONEY,
LOVE, HEALTH AND
HAPPINESS
WITHIN 30 DAYS

VICTORIA FAIRCHILD PORTER

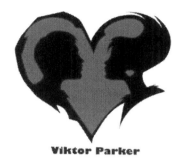

Viktor Parker

Movies to see:

Rebirthing (can find it on You Tube)

Placebo (look for it on You Tube)

Literature:

Ancient Secrets of Fountain of Youth By Peter Kelder

How to make your body produce stem cells By Andrey Levshinov

New drug dramatically increases lifespan, reverses aging By Stephen Morgan

Russian scientist says he is stronger and healthier after injecting himself with 'eternal life' bacteria By Helena Horton

This 122 Year Old Woman Has the Most Important Secret To A Life Of Longevity by Dr. Bruce King

Village in China Holds Oldest, Healthiest People in the World. This is Their Secret by Christina Sarich

Novel antioxidant makes old arteries seem young again, study shows Source: University of Colorado at Boulder

Hormone That Reverses Cell Aging in Humans Identified By Worldhealth

Journal Science Translational Medicine

Mutations Found In 115 Year Old Woman's Blood Could Help Unlock Secrets of Aging by Justine Alford

Researchers may have discovered fountain of youth by reversing aging in human cells by Eric Mack

10 Years Younger By Klaus Oberbeil

Scientists just found a fix for wrinkles By Molly Shea

The FASEB Journal: "Transient delivery of modified mRNA encoding TERT rapidly extends telomeres in human cells"

Top 10 Foods that Age You - Eat These Foods at Your Own Risk by Kellie Oliver

6 Ways to burn Your Belly fat By Jennifer Cohen

Anti-Aging Research Science Genetics in Disease Mechanisms of Aging

Younger Skin Through Exercise By Gretchen Reynolds

By IBTimes Staff Reporter New York PR Newswire

San Medica International by Andrea Perry, femail.co.uk

New research challenges Harvard group's theory that blood from young mice reverses aging

Saturated Fats Damage Health by Promoting Inflammation in Diet Immune System Inflammation

Modern medicine could add 10 years to your lifespan by Zachary D There's Only One Person Alive Born in the 1800s — And Her Diet Is Incredible By Alex Orlov avies Boren

Three-Step Strategy to Reverse Mitochondrial Aging By Michael Downey

Scientists accidentally stop skin aging in mice! By Ryan Whitwam

World's oldest man discovered' Documents claim pensioner is 145 years old By Jack Fenwick

Why Avocados are the Most Unique Antiaging Food by Anya Vien

"Biology of Belief","Spontaneous Evolution" by Bruce Lipton, PhD

Ian Sample, the Guardian (The Long Read)

Confirmed by science: You really can change your DNA - and here's how by Carolanne Wright

Village in China Holds Oldest, Healthiest People in the World. This is Their Secret by Christina Sarich

The Best brain possible with Debbie Hampton

"L-arginine Could Be A Magic Bullet In Your Anti-Aging Arsenal" by Sellers Paradise

Living the longest – indigenous Brazilian celebrates 121st birthday by Surival international

Azerbaijan's Legendary Centenarian Shirali Muslimov Story by Marcus Hopkins Solving the mystery of aging: Longevity gene makes

Hydra immortal and humans grow older Christian-Albrechts-Universitaet zu Kiel

'Indy' gene may be Holy Grail for longevity By Roger Highfield

"Food habits that age you" By Catherine Guthrie

Advanced Glycation End Products By Lori Zanteson Today's Dietitian

11 nutrition lies that vegans will tell you

A secret of anti-aging By Stephanie Relfe & Michael Relfe

101-year-old woman gives birth after successful ovary transplant by Randeep Ramesh

5 Simple Tips to Reduce Skin Pigmentation By Oindrila

The Complete Book of Enzyme Therapy By Dr. Anthony J. Cichoke

Scientists 'REVERSE' menopause: Women who'd not had a period in five years are now menstruating again after their ovaries were rejuvenated By Anna Hodgekiss

Kaya Kalpa: Life Extension and Immortality By Andrea Pflaumer

Proteolytic Enzymes Reduce Inflammation and Boost Immunity By Dr. Axe

Eradicating mitochondria from cells may reverse aging Written by Honor Whiteman

Scientists extend life by 35 percent in mice by clearing cellular 'litter' by Jessica Firger

11 Nutrition Lies That Vegans Will Tell You by Kris Gunnars, Authority

10 Best Natural Methods to Remove Turkey Wattle Neck and Tighten Loose Sagging Neck Skin Tighten Loose Sagging Neck Skin and Remove Turkey Wattle Neck

How to get rid of wrinkles naturally by Siski Green

Reverse, Slow Aging and Prevent Disease With The Humble Sprout! By Dawn Vezie

The Most Powerful Natural Antioxidant Discovered to Date - Hydroxytyrosol By Karen Lee Richards

Kotaku.com By George Dvorsky

dailymail.co.uk By Will Stewart for Mail online

Mercola.com

wisc.edu brucelipton.com

Natural News

Science daily

Oprah.com

Natural Society

survincity.com

healthandlovepage.com

Sugarstacks.com

Agefoundation.com

Thebestbrainpossible.org

appliedergogenics.blogspot.com

81063097R00083

Made in the USA
Lexington, KY
10 February 2018